The Hidden Architecture

SECRET HEALTH RESET BOOK

What Big Pharma Won't Tell You About
Inflammation, Fatigue, and the True
Path to Healing

Staten House

"Truth isn't loud. But once you hear it, you can't unhear it."

Table of Contents

INTRODUCTION

What if the system isn't broken—but working exactly as designed?
You've probably felt it. The persistent fatigue that sleep doesn't fix. The brain fog that blurs your thinking. The bloating, the low mood, the strange symptoms that get brushed off with a shrug or a prescription. And deep down, a growing feeling that something is wrong—not just with your body, but with the story we've been told about health.

This book was written for people like you. People who are tired of being dismissed, drugged, or sent home with vague advice that never addresses the root cause. People who are smart enough to question a system that profits from managing illness instead of preventing it. People who sense—whether intuitively or through experience—that real healing must come from somewhere deeper.

What you're about to read isn't a conspiracy theory. It's not hype. And it's not another feel-good wellness trend. It's a clear, grounded, evidence-aligned guide to reclaiming control over your own health in a world that benefits from keeping you unwell.

Why This Book Exists

We live in a time when chronic illness is normalized, and true vitality is rare. The medical model has its strengths—especially in emergencies—but it's ill-equipped to deal with the root-level dysfunction that so many people now face: inflammation, metabolic chaos, gut disruption, hormone imbalances, nervous system overload.

Instead of addressing these root causes, we've been sold a cycle of symptom suppression. We're told our suffering is normal. We're handed pills, diets, diagnoses, and distractions—but not clarity, not empowerment, and rarely a path forward that truly works.

This book is here to change that.

What You'll Find Inside

The Secret Health Reset Book is divided into three parts. In **Part I**, you'll uncover the hidden forces—both inside your body and in the systems around you—that are quietly sabotaging your health. From misleading health narratives to environmental toxins and corporate influence, this is the part that opens your eyes and validates what you've likely suspected for years.

In **Part II**, you'll begin the actual reset process. This isn't a 30-day detox or a trendy protocol. It's a realignment—starting with what you eat, how you move, what you believe, and how you relate to your body. We'll walk step by step through practical, powerful changes you can make, grounded in biology and real-world science.

In **Part III**, you'll learn how to sustain those changes. Healing is not a destination—it's a lifestyle. Here, we'll talk about rhythm, nervous system resilience, mindset, food as information, and how to protect your progress in a world that constantly pulls you back toward dysfunction.

A Note on Ethics

This book won't promise miracle cures. It won't ask you to reject medicine. And it won't promote anything unsupported or irresponsible. Every page has been written with care to remain firmly rooted in integrity, practicality, and respect for the complexity of the human body.

But make no mistake: it will challenge the narrative you've been given. It will shine a light on the uncomfortable truths behind how modern illness is created and maintained. And it will show you how to begin again—not by outsourcing your health, but by reclaiming it from the inside out.

You deserve more than symptom management. You deserve clarity. You deserve energy. You deserve to feel like yourself again.

Let's begin the reset.

PART I: The Hidden Crisis

Most people don't wake up thinking their daily routine is harming them. They grab breakfast, scroll their phone, head to work, pick up groceries, maybe squeeze in a workout or some family time before bed. From the outside, it all seems "normal." But beneath this surface of routine lies a deeper, more troubling reality—one that millions of people feel in their bodies but can't quite name.

This part of the book is about naming it.

Because the symptoms so many are quietly struggling with—low energy, anxiety, foggy thinking, unexplained weight gain, persistent bloating, disrupted sleep—aren't random. They're signals. Not just of individual health breakdowns, but of a system-wide crisis we've been trained to overlook.

We live in a culture where feeling "off" is brushed aside, where the solution to every issue is often a pill, a patch, or another product. And while medical advances have done incredible things, the truth is that the system isn't designed for prevention. It's built around management—around keeping symptoms quiet rather than uncovering why they're there in the first place.

Part I pulls back the curtain.

We'll explore how common symptoms are often early warning signs, how the narrative around health has been shaped by profit rather than truth, and how many of the ideas we've been sold—from what "healthy" looks like to how disease develops—are incomplete at best, and misleading at worst.

This is where the reset begins: not with another supplement or hack, but with awareness. The kind that changes how you see your body, your environment, and the forces influencing your choices.

This is not about blame—it's about clarity. Because you deserve to know the truth about your health. And the first step to healing is realizing the system wasn't built to make you well.

Let's uncover what's really going on.

The Silent Saboteurs

Everyday Poisons We Mistake for Normal

If you're like most people, your daily life feels pretty normal. You eat meals labeled "natural" or "heart healthy." You clean your home with familiar brands. You use lotions that promise glowing skin. And you've probably assumed that if something was truly dangerous, it wouldn't be allowed on store shelves.

But the truth is: many of the substances we've come to accept as normal are quietly undermining our health every day.

What makes them so dangerous isn't just their toxicity. It's how familiar they are. These "everyday poisons" don't come with warning labels. They don't look like risk. They've been woven into our routines so seamlessly that we rarely question them—until the symptoms show up.

Fatigue. Brain fog. Hormonal imbalances. Gut distress. Skin issues. Chronic inflammation. We treat these as isolated problems, not realizing they're often the body's alarm bells—warning us about constant low-level exposure to substances it was never designed to process.

Let's start where this toxic load begins for most of us: food.

The Hidden Harm in Our Food

Walk through any grocery store and you'll see shelves lined with bright packaging and health claims. "Low-fat," "immune-boosting," "all-natural." But behind the labels is an uncomfortable truth: much of what we eat today isn't real food—it's industrial product engineered for shelf life, not nourishment.

Refined seed oils, like soybean, corn, and canola, are a prime example. They've been marketed as heart-healthy alternatives to saturated fats, but research increasingly links them to oxidative stress and systemic inflammation. These oils are often extracted with solvents like hexane, then deodorized and bleached before hitting your plate—yet they're used in everything from salad dressings to so-called healthy snacks.

Additives are another silent threat. Emulsifiers, artificial sweeteners, preservatives, and colorants can alter the gut microbiome, disrupt hormone signaling, and contribute to metabolic dysfunction. Some, like certain food dyes and preservatives, are banned in other countries but remain legal in the U.S. thanks to outdated safety reviews and aggressive lobbying.

Even the sugar we consume—especially in its high-fructose corn syrup form—drives fatty liver disease, insulin resistance, and chronic inflammation. Yet it's added to everything from sandwich bread to pasta sauces, often under names we don't recognize.

And then there's "ultra-processed food" as a whole category. These are products designed to bypass your natural satiety signals, hijack dopamine pathways, and keep you eating far beyond hunger. They may not look or taste "toxic," but their effects on cellular health, gut permeability, and systemic inflammation are anything but benign.

A System Designed for Profit, Not Prevention

The question isn't how these ingredients slipped through the cracks—it's how they were deliberately placed into the system.

The food industry is a powerful machine with enormous influence over regulation, research, and even public messaging. Health organizations often rely on industry-funded studies that minimize harm, while government food policies continue to subsidize crops that feed the processed food pipeline.

Meanwhile, the average consumer—trying to eat "clean" and "balanced"—is left navigating a landscape where poison is packaged as progress. The most damaging foods are the most accessible, affordable, and aggressively advertised. And unless you've taken the time to deeply investigate what's in your food, you've likely been exposed to thousands of these substances already.

But food is just the beginning.

While the food industry shapes what ends up on our plates, the chemical burden doesn't stop there. Many of the most harmful toxins are found not in what we eat, but in what we breathe, touch, and surround ourselves with—every single day.

Toxic Products Masquerading as Clean

Let's take cleaning supplies. The smell of "lemon fresh" or "mountain breeze" might signal a clean home, but it often means your air is filled with volatile organic compounds (VOCs). These substances are found in air fresheners, disinfectants, and multipurpose sprays, and many are linked to respiratory irritation, hormone disruption, and even increased cancer risk with long-term exposure.

Fragrances—listed simply as "parfum" or "fragrance" on product labels—can contain hundreds of undisclosed chemicals, including phthalates and synthetic musks. These substances are known endocrine disruptors, meaning they interfere with hormonal function at even low doses.

Then there's plastic. From food packaging to personal care bottles, plastic compounds like BPA (and its replacements, like BPS) can leach into products, especially when heated. These chemicals mimic estrogen and are linked to fertility issues, developmental problems, and metabolic disorders. Even "BPA-free" labels don't guarantee safety—they often just swap one harmful chemical for another untested one.

What We Put on Our Skin Matters

The skin is the body's largest organ—and it absorbs much of what we put on it. Unfortunately, many of the lotions, sunscreens, deodorants, and cosmetics we use daily contain ingredients that would never be allowed in food, yet still enter our bloodstream through dermal absorption.

Parabens, triclosan, oxybenzone, aluminum salts, and formaldehyde-releasing preservatives are just a few of the common culprits. These compounds have been associated with immune disruption, reproductive toxicity, and altered thyroid function.

And because personal care products are so under-regulated, manufacturers are not required to test ingredients for long-term safety before putting them on the market. As a result, consumers are left exposed to a cocktail of low-dose chemicals—many of which haven't been studied in combination but are used together daily for years.

The Invisible Toll of Everyday Life

Beyond the obvious chemical culprits, some of the most insidious toxins are the ones we never think to question.

Blue light exposure from screens disrupts circadian rhythms and suppresses melatonin production, which in turn impairs sleep quality and hormone regulation. Chronic sleep disruption increases risk for everything from metabolic dysfunction to mental health issues.

Chronic stress, too, is a kind of toxin. When cortisol stays elevated due to constant alerts, busy schedules, financial pressure, and social comparison, it weakens the immune system, promotes fat storage, and worsens inflammation. Over time, this can mimic and magnify the effects of environmental toxins—creating a perfect storm for dysfunction.

Even the water we drink, depending on its source, can carry contaminants like lead, chlorine byproducts, PFAS ("forever chemicals"), and pesticide residues. While municipal water is treated for biological safety, chemical safety is often a different story—especially for people with sensitive systems.

Why Awareness Is the First Step to Healing

The goal here is not to instill fear, but to restore clarity.

We've been led to believe that everything we're exposed to must be safe—because if it weren't, someone would've stopped it. But safety regulations are slow to adapt, influenced by industry interests, and often based on outdated science. Most toxins we're exposed to today were never tested in combination with others, nor over decades of cumulative use.

And that's why symptoms like fatigue, brain fog, hormonal issues, anxiety, or skin flare-ups are so often misdiagnosed or dismissed. The body isn't just "breaking down." It's reacting to an environment it was never designed to survive in—one we've normalized without realizing.

But knowledge is power. When you start to recognize where these exposures come from, you gain the ability to shift. You may not be able to control every variable, but you can make smarter choices. You can reduce the burden. And you can give your body a fighting chance to heal.

In the next chapters, we'll explore how to do exactly that. You'll learn how to remove key toxins, reset your environment, and support your body's natural detox pathways—not with hype, but with practical steps backed by real science.

Because what's been sold to us as "normal" is not the same as "safe." And health begins with seeing clearly.

How the System Fails to Protect You

Most people assume that if something is allowed on store shelves or prescribed by a doctor, it must be safe. After all, there are entire institutions—government agencies, health organizations, regulatory bodies—tasked with protecting public health. But what if these systems, the very ones we rely on to keep us safe, aren't actually doing what we think they are?

This chapter isn't about stoking fear. It's about removing the blindfold. Because part of resetting your health isn't just about what you eat or how much you sleep—it's about understanding the environment you're living in, the assumptions you've inherited, and the institutions you've trusted. And most of all, it's about reclaiming your right to ask better questions.

Let's start with a difficult truth: regulation often follows, rather than prevents, harm. Time and time again, substances have been declared safe for public use—only to be banned or restricted decades later after undeniable damage was done. Lead in paint and gasoline. Asbestos in insulation. BPA in plastics. Trans fats in processed foods. Each was once approved and widespread, defended by experts and backed by research—until they weren't.

This pattern isn't a fluke. It's a reflection of a system that moves slowly, that's influenced by corporate interests, and that often requires overwhelming evidence before taking action. In the meantime, you're left exposed.

Take food labeling, for example. Most consumers believe they're protected by nutritional guidelines and ingredient transparency. But labels are often manipulated through loopholes. Manufacturers can hide multiple forms of sugar under different names. "Natural flavors" can contain dozens of synthetic compounds. And a product labeled "healthy" may still be loaded with inflammatory oils, additives, and chemicals that disrupt your gut or hormones.

It's the same with personal care and household products. In many countries, thousands of chemicals are allowed in cosmetics, cleaning sprays, and air fresheners without rigorous long-term testing. And the burden of proof isn't on companies to show something is safe—it's on regulators to prove harm, often after people have already been exposed for years.

Even more concerning is the revolving door between government agencies and the industries they regulate. Former executives from pharmaceutical companies, agrochemical giants, and food conglomerates regularly move into regulatory positions—and vice versa. It creates a culture where profit and policy are tangled together, and where decisions may reflect corporate strategy more than public interest.

Of course, there are brilliant scientists, doctors, and public servants working hard to protect people. But they're doing so within a structure that often prioritizes market stability, political interests, and economic growth over precaution. That's not a conspiracy—it's just how the system is built.

And then there's the influence of research funding. Studies that shape policy and health recommendations are frequently funded by the very companies whose products are being evaluated. This doesn't automatically mean bad science, but it does raise serious concerns about bias. Independent research is often underfunded and underpromoted. Meanwhile, industry-backed studies tend to get more attention, more favorable coverage, and more traction in shaping what gets recommended to the public.

So where does that leave you?

It leaves you in a position of needing to become your own filter. Not a cynic, not a skeptic of all science—but someone who understands the layers of influence behind the information you're given.

This doesn't mean you need to become a full-time investigator. It means you   start   asking:

Who funded this study?

What financial interests might be involved in this recommendation?

Why has something become "normal" despite rising health issues?

When you begin seeing how the system is structured, things that once seemed confusing begin to make more sense. You start noticing how symptoms are treated in isolation instead of addressing root causes. How medications are often prescribed for life, rather than short-term recovery. How public health campaigns rarely talk about prevention beyond surface-level advice. And how entire populations are now chronically inflamed, fatigued, and dependent—not because they're broken, but because the system never prioritized true wellness.

This chapter isn't about pointing fingers. It's about giving you the context to understand why your body may be struggling—and why you're not alone.

Because if you've felt ignored by doctors, confused by conflicting health advice, or ashamed for not feeling better despite "doing everything right," the problem isn't you. It's that you've been trying to thrive in a system that was never designed for it.

The good news? You don't need to burn it all down or go live in a cabin in the woods. You just need to start seeing clearly. That's what this book— and this reset—is about. Not blind rebellion. Not submission. But discernment.

Your body is intelligent. It's constantly trying to adapt, to heal, to protect you—even in an environment filled with noise, toxins, and half-truths. When you start recognizing the factors around you for what they are—not as unchangeable realities but as navigable terrain—you begin to reclaim the power you never really lost.

And that's the point: to wake up from the haze. To stop mistaking chronic symptoms for normal life. And to realize that your health isn't just yours to protect—it's yours to define, on your terms, guided by truth instead of marketing.

Because once you see the system clearly, you no longer expect it to save you. And that's when real healing begins.

But recognizing the system's shortcomings isn't just an intellectual exercise. It has real-world consequences for your daily life—what you eat, what you buy, the questions you ask at the doctor's office, and the way you respond to your own symptoms.

Let's take a step back and look at how the everyday person is shaped by this structure. From a young age, you're conditioned to defer health decisions to authority. You're told the doctor knows best. That side effects are just part of the deal. That symptoms are random, or genetic, or inevitable. And that healing always comes from the outside in—a pill, a shot, a procedure.

This mindset runs deep. And in many cases, it strips you of agency. You start believing that your symptoms are mysteries too complex for you to understand. That discomfort is just something to manage. That feeling tired, bloated, or anxious all the time is just "modern life." But what if your body is trying to communicate something? What if those signals aren't random— but messages?

The system, as it exists, is not built to empower you to explore those messages. It's structured to compartmentalize and intervene. You see one

16

specialist for digestion, another for hormones, another for mood—and each operates in a silo. Rarely does someone step back to ask how your food, your environment, your stress, and your lifestyle intersect.

This fragmentation isn't just inefficient. It's misleading. It teaches people to separate their bodies into disconnected parts rather than seeing the full, intelligent system that it is. It reinforces the idea that you need external management, not internal alignment. And so, over time, the person who once intuitively knew what foods made them feel off or what situations spiked their anxiety becomes someone who no longer trusts their own perception.

The consequences aren't just physical. They're emotional, too. Feeling ignored, dismissed, or misunderstood by a medical provider—especially when your symptoms are real but don't fit into a neat diagnostic box—can leave lasting scars. You start second-guessing yourself. You wonder if it really is all in your head. And in that doubt, your power quietly slips away.

To be clear, this isn't about villainizing healthcare professionals. Most enter the field with a deep desire to help. But they are trained within the same system we're examining—a system that often prioritizes treatment over prevention, speed over listening, and standardization over personalization.

And yet, this is where your opportunity lies. Because once you see the limits of the model, you're no longer confined by it. You can begin to take ownership—not in a reactionary, anti-science way, but in a grounded, informed, and proactive way. You can begin to explore how food, movement, rest, nervous system balance, emotional health, and connection all contribute to real healing.

You don't need a medical degree to start tuning into your body. You don't need to reject everything conventional medicine offers. You just need to stop outsourcing the entirety of your health to systems that were never designed for full human flourishing. Use what serves you. Question what doesn't. And above all, don't confuse being compliant with being well.

The truth is, systems are slow to change. But individuals can change quickly. And when enough individuals shift—asking better questions, demanding better options, stepping into their own authority—systems eventually follow. But it starts small. It starts with you.

With each chapter of this book, you'll gain a clearer understanding of how to interpret your symptoms, reset your body's natural rhythm, and reconnect with the signals that have always been there—just waiting to be heard. You'll learn how to spot the influences that have kept you stuck and how to gently but powerfully remove what's been weighing your health down.

This isn't about becoming your own doctor. It's about becoming your own advocate. It's about knowing enough to collaborate, to challenge respectfully, and to take the lead in your own wellness journey.

Because in the end, your greatest protection isn't a perfect system—it's awareness, discernment, and your willingness to question the status quo in pursuit of something better.

You are not broken. You are not crazy. You're waking up.

And that changes everything.

The Symptoms You've Been Taught to Ignore

You wake up tired, even after a full night's sleep. You feel bloated after meals, your skin acts up for no clear reason, and your mood swings hit harder than you'd like to admit. Maybe your joints ache in the morning or your mind feels foggy by mid-afternoon. But you keep going. You tell yourself it's stress. Or age. Or hormones. Or just life.

These symptoms—persistent, subtle, and often dismissed—are exactly the ones we've been conditioned to ignore. We're taught to normalize them. Power through. Blame ourselves. Wait until they become serious enough to "deserve" medical attention.

In today's fast-paced world, chronic discomfort has become a kind of background noise. Everyone seems to be exhausted or anxious or slightly unwell, so we assume it's just the way things are. But what if these symptoms are not random? What if they're actually your body's early warning system? Signals that something is out of balance?

Here's the hard truth: the modern health system often overlooks these quieter symptoms because they don't fit neatly into a diagnosis—or because addressing them doesn't fit the speed and structure of conventional care. A ten-minute appointment isn't long enough to explore the root cause of your digestive issues or fatigue. It's enough time to prescribe an antacid or an antidepressant, not to understand your life.

And so you learn to silence your body's messages. You learn to suppress instead of listen. You treat symptoms like problems to get rid of, rather than invitations to go deeper.

This doesn't mean the system is entirely broken. It means it's built for acute care, not chronic complexity. It's designed to intervene in crisis, not to investigate nuance. And for many people, that leaves a massive gap between "not sick" and "truly well."

That's the space where most of us live. Not in the ICU, but not thriving either. Functioning, but flat. Getting by, but not feeling whole. And in that in-between, the body is constantly speaking. It whispers first. If ignored, it starts to shout.

Take fatigue. Not just the kind that comes from one late night, but the relentless tiredness that sleep doesn't fix. It could be a sign of nutrient deficiencies, poor mitochondrial function, imbalanced blood sugar, chronic inflammation, or unresolved emotional stress. But instead of investigating, we pour another cup of coffee. We call ourselves lazy. We keep pushing.

Or consider brain fog. That frustrating inability to focus, recall words, or stay mentally sharp. It's often brushed off as aging or distraction. But it could stem from gut imbalances, poor detoxification, food sensitivities, or sleep dysregulation. Still, how often do we stop and ask what our fog might be trying to tell us?

The same goes for skin issues, bloating, mood swings, hormonal irregularities, or recurring aches. These are not random events. They are part of a conversation your body is trying to have with you.

The problem is that most of us were never taught to speak the body's language. We were taught to wait for a crisis—or to seek reassurance that "everything looks fine" on a blood test. And so, we override. We take medications to mute symptoms without asking what caused them in the first place.

But what if we stopped seeing these symptoms as annoyances or evidence of personal failure? What if we treated them as intelligent signals—indicators that something in our environment, our lifestyle, or even our beliefs is misaligned with health?

One of the biggest shifts in modern wellness comes when we reframe symptoms not as enemies, but as messengers. That mild but persistent headache? It might be about more than hydration. That anxiety spike at 3 p.m.? Maybe your blood sugar is on a roller coaster. That PMS that wipes you out for a week? It could point to endocrine disruption, not "just how it is to be a woman."

Our culture has normalized the idea that these experiences are simply part of adulthood. But they're not. They're part of a widespread systemic dysfunction—nutritional gaps, sleep deprivation, endocrine disruption, overexposure to chemicals, and emotional dysregulation—all of which are increasingly common in our modern environment.

Unfortunately, these signs are usually met with superficial fixes. Quick answers. A prescription, a supplement, a "biohack." And while some of these tools can help, they're often offered without the deeper context: Why is this happening in the first place? What pattern is your body trying to reveal?

True health begins when we learn to decode that pattern. It's about noticing that your anxiety spikes after certain foods—or that your skin clears up when you finally sleep well. It's about paying attention to the gut feeling (literally) that something isn't sitting right. It's about trusting that your body wants to heal—and is constantly trying to guide you toward balance, even if the path isn't obvious.

This means building a relationship with your symptoms instead of fighting them. It means slowing down enough to ask, "What might this be about?" rather than reaching for the fastest fix. It's not always convenient. And it doesn't always lead to immediate relief. But it does lead to deeper healing—the kind that builds resilience, clarity, and self-trust.

For example, say you're dealing with constant bloating. You've tried cutting out dairy and gluten. You've taken probiotics. Nothing helps for long. Instead of giving up or assuming "that's just how my body is," the new question becomes: what's still inflaming my gut? Is it my stress levels? My meal timing? The way I eat—rushed and distracted, rather than slow and present?

Or maybe you've noticed your mood crashing mid-cycle, every month. The conventional system may offer antidepressants or birth control. But a deeper lens asks: is my liver clearing estrogen efficiently? Is my nutrition supporting hormonal balance? Are my emotions being suppressed and showing up in my body?

These questions don't always yield simple answers. But they open the door to a much more empowered conversation with your health. And that's what this reset is really about—not just eliminating discomfort, but reconnecting with the signals your body is constantly sending.

This doesn't mean you ignore medical advice. It doesn't mean symptoms are always spiritual or psychological. It means you recognize the limitations of a model that only reacts when things go catastrophically wrong. And you choose to get curious earlier.

You learn to see patterns in your symptoms, to track your cycles, to experiment with changes, to ask better questions. And slowly, you begin to reclaim the wisdom that's been there all along.

Because healing isn't about perfection or the absence of all symptoms. It's about creating enough space and stability in your system that when a symptom shows up, you know how to listen. You know how to respond. You know how to support yourself.

And that shift—from suppression to collaboration—is one of the most powerful steps on the path to true health.

Let's begin.

Why You Still Feel Sick

The False Health Narrative

For decades, we've been taught a story about health that feels reassuring on the surface: that our bodies are largely unpredictable machines, that illness strikes randomly, and that the best we can do is manage symptoms with expert help and modern pharmaceuticals. It's a comforting idea in its simplicity—but it's not the truth.

This narrative, repeated across media, medicine, and education, subtly trains us to give our authority away. If you feel unwell, the solution lies "out there"—in a pill, a procedure, or a specialist with letters after their name. You're told not to worry about the root cause. Just patch it up and move on.

But here's the quiet part that rarely gets said aloud: this model wasn't designed to make you well. It was designed to make you compliant.

That may sound harsh. But look at the incentives. In a system where profit depends on recurring treatments, not prevention, there's little room to address the actual causes of chronic illness—environmental toxins, nutrient-depleted food, overprescribed medications, emotional trauma, and systemic stress. These issues aren't easy to medicate. They require long-term change, awareness, and participation from the individual. That's not a great business model.

So instead, we've been sold a more convenient version of reality. One that suggests inflammation, fatigue, autoimmune flares, mood disorders, and hormonal chaos are simply part of modern life. One where each of these symptoms is isolated, labeled, and medicated—never investigated as part of a larger picture.

This is the false health narrative: a system of beliefs that keeps you disconnected from your body, convinced that your suffering is just how it has to be.

And it's everywhere. You see it in commercials telling you that bloating is normal. In ads that sell antidepressants without asking what's causing the depression. In wellness products that promise transformation without addressing what's actually broken in your lifestyle or environment.

Even well-meaning professionals can reinforce the narrative. When your labs are "normal," but you still feel off, you might be told it's in your head. When you ask about food sensitivities, you may be dismissed. When you suspect stress is affecting your hormones, you're advised to "relax." The system doesn't know how to deal with complexity. So it simplifies. It fragments. It overlooks.

But your body is not fragmented. Your symptoms aren't isolated glitches. They're part of a holistic language—a system of feedback that reflects how your physical, emotional, and environmental inputs are interacting.

Once you begin to decode that system, the story changes. You stop seeing yourself as broken. You start recognizing the intelligence beneath your symptoms. And you begin to understand just how much power you actually have.

The real danger of the false narrative isn't just that it misguides people—it's that it erodes self-trust. It teaches you to override your instincts. To doubt your experience. To outsource your wellness entirely.

This is why so many people live for years in a kind of quiet health purgatory. They're not "sick enough" to warrant urgent intervention, but they're not truly well either. They're surviving—but disconnected, tired, inflamed, anxious, and unsure why nothing seems to work.

They've followed the rules. Eaten low-fat. Slept (sometimes). Exercised (a bit). Taken the medications. And yet... the fog never lifts. The energy never returns. The weight never drops. The cycle continues.

It's not because they've failed. It's because they've been handed a framework that was never designed to produce true health in the first place. The narrative fails because it's built on fragmentation—of knowledge, of systems, and most dangerously, of self-awareness. You're expected to see your gut as separate from your brain, your mood as separate from your hormones, your food as separate from your medicine. But nothing in nature works this way. Your body certainly doesn't.

Once you recognize that truth, the cracks in the story become obvious. You begin to question why a system that claims to care about health rarely speaks about clean water, nutritious food, movement, rest, sunlight, or emotional processing. You begin to notice how quick it is to offer suppression—of pain, of emotion, of symptoms—without asking what those experiences are trying to reveal.

And you may start to see something even more unsettling: how your disempowerment serves a larger design. Because the more disconnected you are from your body's wisdom, the easier it is to market solutions to you. The more you distrust your own signals, the more you'll rely on authority figures to interpret them for you. The less agency you have, the more compliant you become.

This isn't a conspiracy—it's a consequence. Of a system designed for volume, speed, and profit, not nuance, prevention, or true healing.

But the good news is this: once you see it, you can step out of it.

Reclaiming your health means reclaiming your narrative. It means no longer seeing your symptoms as random or meaningless. It means remembering that your body is a dynamic, adaptive, deeply intelligent system that's always trying to protect you—even when it's inflamed, exhausted, or out of balance.

This doesn't mean you should reject all of conventional medicine. There are brilliant doctors doing vital work, and acute care medicine saves lives every day. But it does mean that you must begin to take responsibility for asking the deeper questions. Why am I experiencing this? What is my body responding to? What's the root, not just the surface?

It also means being willing to hold two truths at once: that you've likely been misled, and that you still hold the power to reset. That your suffering is valid, and that healing is possible. That the system may have failed you, but you don't have to keep failing yourself.

This is where your health journey truly begins—not with a new pill or protocol, but with a shift in mindset. A willingness to listen again. To your body. To your intuition. To the subtle ways your life and environment are either nourishing or depleting you.

It's an unlearning as much as it is a learning. You unlearn the belief that health is something you outsource. You unlearn the idea that you're powerless. You unlearn the myth that being "fine" is the best you can hope for.

And in that space, something new opens up. A quiet but steady clarity. A deep reconnection. A sense that your body has been waiting all along for you to come back home.

Because healing isn't about perfection. It's about partnership. With your body. With your choices. With the truth.

And once you begin to live from that place, the false health narrative loses its grip. You no longer need to believe it—because you're living the proof that something better is possible.

That's not a theory. That's not hype. That's lived experience—yours, and that of countless others who have decided to stop waiting for the system to fix them and instead began the work of truly restoring themselves.

The story changes now. And you get to be the one who rewrites it.

From Fatigue to Fog: What Your Body Is Telling You

It often starts subtly. You hit the snooze button more times than usual. You find yourself staring blankly at the same paragraph, unable to absorb it. You walk into a room and forget why you're there. You chalk it up to stress, age, poor sleep—but deep down, something doesn't feel quite right.

Fatigue and brain fog are so common that many people no longer see them as symptoms. They're brushed off as normal parts of a busy, modern life. But just because something is common doesn't make it normal. And when your body is whispering through exhaustion and mental haze, it's not asking for caffeine or motivation. It's sending a message.

Your energy is a currency—and fatigue is your body's way of telling you it's overspent.

We often equate tiredness with effort, assuming that if we're exhausted, we must have worked hard. But fatigue without a clear cause is something different. It's not just about not getting enough sleep—it's about how your body is processing everything it's exposed to: the food you eat, the air you breathe, the stress you carry, the screens you stare at, and the low-grade inflammation simmering beneath it all.

And brain fog—this subtle but deeply disruptive symptom—goes hand-in-hand with fatigue. You may feel like your brain is wrapped in cotton. Words slip away. Focus scatters. You lose the thread of conversations, misplace items, feel emotionally flat or easily overwhelmed. These aren't just quirks of personality or signs of getting older. They're signs of imbalance.

One of the most common culprits? Blood sugar dysregulation. When your meals are built around processed carbs and sugar, and you're riding the wave of spikes and crashes all day, your brain pays the price. Every crash pulls you into that hazy, sluggish place where thoughts feel heavy and effortful. And the more this cycle repeats, the more normal it feels—until you forget what clarity actually feels like.

Hormonal shifts also play a powerful role. Cortisol, your stress hormone, is meant to rise in the morning to get you going and fall at night so you can rest. But in chronic stress, this rhythm breaks down. You may feel wired but tired, struggling to wind down even when you're exhausted. Or you may crash in the afternoon and reach for sugar or caffeine to push through, only to lie awake at night, wondering why your body won't cooperate.

Meanwhile, inflammation creates another layer of interference. When your immune system is constantly activated—whether from hidden infections, gut imbalances, or environmental toxins—it uses up a huge amount of energy. That leaves less for basic tasks like clear thinking, memory, or sustained physical output. Your body may be fighting a battle you're not even aware of, and fatigue is its white flag.

But perhaps one of the most overlooked contributors to both fatigue and brain fog is emotional and energetic overload. If you're constantly filtering noise, managing others' expectations, and living in a state of low-grade overwhelm, your nervous system never truly gets a break. Over time, that constant demand drains your vitality, leaving you feeling detached, numb, or flat.

This isn't your fault. Most of us were never taught to recognize these signals as valid, let alone important. We're told to push through, hustle harder, drink more coffee, or "think positively." But when you override the body's signals long enough, it stops whispering—and starts screaming.

And yet, these symptoms are not the problem—they are the body's attempt to solve the problem.

They are your invitation to pause. To look deeper. To ask: What am I really running on? What am I really ignoring? What does my body need that I haven't been giving it?

We'll explore that next. Because when you start listening to what fatigue and fog are truly saying, you begin to uncover the root—and that's where real energy comes from. Not from stimulants or hacks, but from alignment. From healing. From restoring the systems that keep you whole.

Let's start by understanding the biology beneath these signals.

When we look beneath the surface of fatigue and brain fog, we begin to see how deeply interconnected our body's systems really are. These aren't isolated malfunctions. They're downstream effects of a larger imbalance—a signal that your body is stuck in survival mode rather than operating from a place of ease, repair, and vitality.

Start with your mitochondria—the energy factories in your cells. These tiny organelles are responsible for producing the energy that powers everything you do, from muscle contractions to thought processes. But they are exquisitely sensitive to stressors. Exposure to toxins (like pesticides or mold), nutrient deficiencies, inflammation, and even emotional stress can all impair mitochondrial function. When your mitochondria are sluggish, *you* feel sluggish. Your body quite literally can't keep up with what you're asking of it.

The gut plays a major role here too. If the lining of your intestines becomes compromised—a condition often referred to as "leaky gut"—it can allow inflammatory molecules to enter the bloodstream, triggering immune reactions and clouding mental clarity. Add to that the fact that gut bacteria help produce neurotransmitters like serotonin, dopamine, and GABA, and it becomes obvious that gut health is central to how we think, feel, and function. A compromised gut isn't just a digestive issue; it's a neurological one, a hormonal one, and an energy one.

Speaking of hormones, let's not ignore thyroid function. Even subtle imbalances in your thyroid can profoundly impact your energy and cognition. And unfortunately, many people with thyroid dysfunction are told their labs are "normal" when symptoms clearly persist. Conventional testing often misses nuanced issues—like poor conversion of T4 to T3, or the presence of thyroid antibodies indicating autoimmunity. You can be clinically "fine" on paper but feel anything but fine in real life.

Sleep is another piece of the puzzle. Quality sleep is not just about quantity; it's about the body's ability to reach deep, restorative stages. Things like sleep apnea, nighttime blood sugar dips, EMF exposure, and poor sleep hygiene can all interfere with this process, leaving you groggy no matter how many hours you log. And if your nervous system is stuck in a sympathetic (fight-or-flight) state, even your rest isn't truly restful.

But perhaps the most important shift comes from realizing that chronic fatigue and mental fog are not signs that you're broken. They're signs that your body is *still trying*. Still adapting. Still doing its best to protect you with the resources it has.

That shift in perspective—seeing your symptoms as signals rather than failures—can change everything. Instead of blaming yourself or feeling defeated, you begin to approach healing with curiosity and compassion. You ask, "What's missing?" rather than "What's wrong with me?" And more often than not, the answers are there, waiting in plain sight.

Maybe it's that your meals lack the micronutrients your cells need. Maybe you've been surviving on stimulants and adrenaline for too long. Maybe your environment is too loud, your relationships too draining, your boundaries too porous. Maybe you haven't truly *stopped* in years.

When you start removing the things that deplete you—and adding the things that replenish—you begin to feel the fog lift. Not all at once, and not in some perfect linear path. But gradually, steadily, you reclaim access to your own clarity.

Clarity isn't just about cognition. It's about knowing what matters. About being able to feel again. About reconnecting with your own internal signals so that you no longer need to outsource your wellbeing to apps, pills, or protocols.

This chapter isn't about blaming the system or glorifying suffering. It's about truth-telling. About shining a light on what so many people feel in silence, and reminding you that your experience is valid.

You are not lazy. You are not weak. You are not imagining things.

Your body is speaking. The question is—are you ready to listen?

Because once you do, you'll discover something powerful: beneath the fatigue, beneath the fog, there's a resilient intelligence that's always been guiding you home. And that's where the reset truly begins.

When Doctors Say 'It's in Your Head'

There's a moment many people will never forget. You sit in the sterile office under fluorescent lights, trying to explain the weight you've been carrying—the fatigue that won't lift, the brain fog that makes simple tasks feel impossible, the pain that moves around your body like a shape-shifter. And then the doctor looks up from their clipboard and says it: *"Your tests are normal. It might be stress. Maybe it's in your head."*

It's a sentence that lands like a gut punch. On the surface, it might sound benign—even rational. But to someone who has been struggling, searching for answers, and questioning their own sanity, it's deeply invalidating. It suggests that your suffering isn't real unless it can be measured, scanned, or reduced to a number in a lab report.

This experience isn't rare. In fact, it's far more common than many realize, particularly for women, for people with complex or chronic conditions, and for those whose symptoms don't fit neatly into diagnostic categories. Instead of curiosity, they're met with dismissal. Instead of investigation, they're offered a prescription for antidepressants—or worse, a subtle insinuation that they're exaggerating.

But let's be clear: this isn't always the fault of individual doctors. Most are doing their best within a system that trains them to treat disease as a binary: present or not, measurable or not, fixable or not. Medical education prioritizes pathology over prevention, test results over lived experience, and clear diagnoses over nuance. The system rewards speed and certainty, not deep listening or complexity.

So when your lab tests come back within the "normal" range, your story often becomes inconvenient. The absence of a clear cause becomes a reason to stop asking questions. And the result? Countless people are left navigating real, life-disrupting symptoms without validation, support, or a path forward.

Here's the deeper problem: by telling someone "it's in your head," we ignore the very real interplay between mind and body. Yes, stress, trauma, and emotional repression can have physiological effects. But that doesn't mean the symptoms are *imagined*. They're embodied. They manifest through immune dysfunction, hormonal imbalance, nervous system dysregulation, and cellular exhaustion.

In fact, neuroscience and psychoneuroimmunology (the study of how thoughts and emotions impact immune function) have shown us again and again: your mental and emotional state is inseparable from your physical health. The brain doesn't sit in a vacuum. It's in constant conversation with the gut, the heart, the liver, and every other system in your body. So when doctors dismiss symptoms as "just stress," they're not wrong in noting a connection—but they're missing the point entirely.

Because the real question isn't whether your symptoms are influenced by stress. The question is: *why* is your body stuck in stress physiology in the first place? What environments, traumas, deficiencies, toxins, or imbalances are keeping your system on high alert? What's the root, not just the result?

We also have to acknowledge how trauma complicates this picture. People who've experienced emotional or physical trauma—especially in childhood—often develop nervous systems that are hypervigilant. Their bodies learn to survive, to endure, to suppress. And over time, that chronic state of internal tension becomes a breeding ground for inflammation, autoimmunity, and burnout.

At this point in the conversation, we need to pause and reframe the narrative—not just for patients, but for practitioners too.

What if we stopped treating the phrase "it's in your head" as a dismissal and instead used it as a doorway to deeper understanding? What if, instead of being shorthand for "you're imagining it," it became an invitation to look at the integrated, layered systems of the human experience—nervous, endocrine, immune, and emotional—all working together, often below conscious awareness?

There's growing recognition among functional and integrative practitioners that symptoms are messengers, not nuisances to be suppressed. Fatigue, anxiety, brain fog, skin eruptions, or gut discomfort—they're not random. They're not psychological flaws or weaknesses. They are communication. They're your body's attempt to say something isn't right, something is too much, something needs care or change.

But the mainstream medical model often lacks the framework to interpret those signals unless they fit into a well-established diagnostic code. Insurance doesn't reimburse for "something feels off." And most doctors don't have the time—let alone the training—to unpack the root causes behind vague or systemic symptoms. So patients are sent home with a pat on the back, a printout about managing stress, or a prescription they never really wanted.

That lack of validation becomes its own form of harm. Over time, people stop trusting their bodies. They start believing that they're dramatic, broken, or weak. They may even stop talking about their symptoms altogether, resigned to the idea that no one will believe them or that nothing can help. This quiet erosion of self-trust is one of the most dangerous consequences of the "it's in your head" narrative. It silences intuition. It separates people from the wisdom of their own bodies.

What we need is a shift—from reductionism to connection, from symptom suppression to root-cause exploration. This shift doesn't mean rejecting modern medicine. It means demanding more of it. It means building a healthcare culture that values patient experience, that listens without rushing, that recognizes the overlap between emotional pain and physical manifestation, without conflating the two or invalidating either.

It also means returning agency to the individual. Because here's the truth: even when the system fails to validate your pain, that pain is still real. And you still deserve to be well. Healing doesn't always start with a diagnosis—it often begins with believing yourself.

You may have to be the one who asks the harder questions. Who digs into your environment, your food, your sleep, your history, your exposure to chronic stress or trauma. Who looks beyond lab ranges and into how you *actually* feel, day to day. That kind of self-investigation is a brave act—and it's often what opens the door to genuine healing.

If your body is speaking, even in ways that seem inconvenient or confusing, the message matters. The body doesn't lie. It may whisper for a while, then raise its voice, and eventually scream if it's ignored long enough. But always, it speaks in truth.

So if you've been told "it's in your head," let that be your signal—not to doubt yourself, but to dig deeper. To find practitioners who treat you as a whole person, not just a puzzle of symptoms. To educate yourself, to reconnect with your intuition, and to reclaim the narrative around your health.

You are not fragile. You are not imagining it. You are not a problem to be fixed. You are a whole being, doing your best in a system that often overlooks complexity in favor of convenience.

33

Let this chapter be a turning point. Not the end of your search for answers—but the beginning of your return to trust, clarity, and truth. Because the real story isn't that your symptoms are "in your head." The real story is that they're in your body—and your body is worth listening to. Always.

The Conspiracy of Convenience

Profits Over Prevention

When we imagine healthcare, we often picture doctors in white coats, lifesaving surgeries, and scientific breakthroughs that promise better lives. And in many ways, these things are true. Modern medicine has made incredible strides. But underneath the image, there's another, more uncomfortable reality—one that quietly influences nearly every aspect of how health is managed, treated, and discussed in the modern world.

That reality is this: our health system is not primarily built to keep us well. It's built to manage illness in ways that generate profit.

This isn't a conspiracy theory. It's economics. Healthcare is one of the largest industries in the world. In the U.S. alone, it accounts for over $4 trillion annually. That kind of money doesn't come from people being vibrantly healthy. It comes from people who stay stuck in cycles of chronic symptoms, ongoing treatments, recurring prescriptions, and delayed diagnoses.

The system thrives when people are sick enough to need care—but not necessarily sick enough to demand drastic intervention. Chronic fatigue, digestive issues, brain fog, anxiety, hormone imbalances, blood sugar instability—these are the goldmine conditions. Common enough to be widespread. Complex enough to require multiple appointments, tests, and prescriptions. But elusive enough to never reach resolution.

Preventing these conditions—truly preventing them—would threaten an enormous revenue stream.

This is why prevention is rarely the focus. Sure, public health campaigns might tell you to move more, eat your vegetables, or stop smoking. But the deeper, more systemic issues—like environmental toxins, ultra-processed food supply chains, and the unchecked marketing of pharmaceuticals—are rarely addressed at their root.

Because when prevention works, products don't sell.

Consider how much easier it is to prescribe a statin for cholesterol than to help a patient overhaul their lifestyle and nutrition habits. Or how quickly antidepressants are offered, compared to in-depth screenings for trauma, sleep quality, blood sugar dysregulation, or inflammation. This isn't about blaming doctors—most of them genuinely want to help. But they operate within a system that rewards speed, standardization, and pharmaceutical compliance, not root-cause resolution.

The pharmaceutical industry, in particular, is not incentivized to make people well. Its model is built on lifelong customers. A pill you take forever is far more profitable than one you only need for a month. A condition that requires constant monitoring, refills, and specialist visits is far more lucrative than one that's resolved through food, movement, stress reduction, and detoxification.

And so, treatments are pushed. Side effects are minimized. Alternatives are sidelined.

Even research is shaped by this model. Studies that don't promise a patentable outcome often go unfunded. Nutritional interventions, environmental exposures, or holistic approaches are underrepresented in the literature—not necessarily because they don't work, but because there's no billion-dollar upside in validating them.

The result is a system that confuses maintenance with healing. That teaches patients to manage symptoms, but rarely to question where those symptoms came from in the first place. That tells people their conditions are "genetic" or "age-related" or simply "bad luck," when in reality, many of these outcomes are influenced by modifiable factors—factors we're rarely educated about.

The tension between profit and prevention becomes even more clear when you look at how information is shared with the public. Large food corporations fund studies that conveniently absolve their products. Pharmaceutical companies advertise directly to consumers, often glossing over side effects while promising a quick fix. And social media platforms increasingly censor or bury content that challenges the dominant medical narratives, regardless of how grounded it may be in emerging science or lived experience.

This leaves patients confused, overwhelmed, and dependent.

When the system is structured around treatment instead of healing, it doesn't just shape how medicine is practiced—it subtly shapes what we believe about our bodies.

Many people have been conditioned to see their symptoms as flaws, rather than messages. They've learned to suppress discomfort instead of exploring it. When fatigue hits, the solution is caffeine. When sleep suffers, it's melatonin or a prescription. When digestion is off, there's a supplement or a pill. The question rarely becomes: "Why is my body asking for help?" Instead, it becomes: "How can I shut this down fast so I can keep going?"

This mentality, while understandable in a fast-paced world, is a direct result of a system that teaches us to silence symptoms instead of resolving their root causes. It's profitable to have people who are barely functioning. It's profitable to frame health as something too complicated for the average person to understand—something that requires endless specialists and protocols. And it's profitable to convince people that wellness can only be achieved through products, subscriptions, and lifelong regimens.

But true prevention is not a product. It's not flashy. And often, it doesn't make headlines. It looks like basic, unglamorous choices repeated daily. Eating whole, unprocessed food. Moving regularly. Sleeping deeply. Limiting exposure to known toxins. Managing stress. Supporting the body's detox pathways. None of this can be patented, and yet, it's often more powerful than any pill.

Unfortunately, many of these preventive foundations have been eroded by the very industries that profit when they break down. Our food is stripped of nutrients and laced with additives. Our water carries residues of industrial runoff and pharmaceuticals. Our homes are filled with synthetic chemicals. Even the air we breathe, especially indoors, is often more polluted than we realize. All of this adds up, slowly taxing the body over time—until chronic symptoms emerge.

By the time someone starts to feel "off," the default path is usually a medical one. Labs, referrals, prescriptions. It's not that these tools don't have a place—they absolutely do. But when they're the only path offered, we lose something vital: the power to intervene before illness takes root. We lose agency.

And this is where the narrative must change. Reclaiming health doesn't start with fighting the system head-on. It starts with awareness. With recognizing the patterns that have shaped our beliefs. With understanding how marketing, policy, and profit have influenced what we accept as "normal."

Because what's considered normal today—chronic fatigue, bloating, anxiety, joint pain, skin issues, hormonal chaos—is not actually normal. It's just common. And common does not mean inevitable.

When we start to question these patterns, something shifts. We stop blaming ourselves for not feeling well. We stop internalizing the idea that our suffering is just part of life or aging or being "too sensitive." We begin to see our symptoms not as nuisances to medicate away, but as early signals—whispers from the body asking for attention.

From this place, prevention becomes powerful again. Not the watered-down version that says "eat healthy" in vague terms, but the kind that asks you to take ownership of your environment, your inputs, your routines. The kind that says your health is not a mystery—it's a reflection of what you're exposed to, what you absorb, and how your body is supported in adapting to it all.

That's not always an easy path. It requires effort, discernment, and sometimes swimming against the current of mainstream advice. But it's also deeply empowering. Because when you stop outsourcing your wellness to a system that wasn't built to see you thrive, you reclaim your right to feel well—not just "not sick," but truly vibrant.

Profits may still drive the system. But awareness can drive change. And it starts with individuals who refuse to accept dysfunction as their baseline. It starts with you.

Suppressed Science and Censored Truth

It's easy to believe that medical science is purely objective—that data rises to the surface because it's true, and treatments are approved because they work. But history tells a different story. Again and again, discoveries that could have transformed health outcomes were ignored, discredited, or buried—not because they were wrong, but because they were inconvenient. Science, for all its brilliance, doesn't exist in a vacuum. It lives within systems shaped by funding, politics, power, and profit. And when a study threatens to disrupt a profitable narrative—one that benefits pharmaceutical companies, food conglomerates, or regulatory agencies—it often gets sidelined.

Some of the world's greatest breakthroughs have come not from the mainstream, but from fringe thinkers who challenged dominant paradigms. Yet too often, those voices were silenced. Not because they lacked evidence, but because their findings posed a threat to the status quo. A supplement that outperforms a drug, a food-based protocol that reverses symptoms, or a chemical shown to disrupt hormones—these are not just scientific curiosities. They're liabilities in a marketplace that thrives on illness, not wellness.

Consider how many researchers have struggled to get funding for studies that aren't patentable. Whole-food interventions, mindfulness, environmental detoxification—these approaches don't generate billion-dollar returns, so they often don't attract institutional support. The result? A body of medical literature that's skewed toward what can be monetized.

And then there's the censorship—more subtle, but no less damaging. A study might be published, but in a low-impact journal with little media attention. A respected doctor may raise concerns about overprescription, only to be discredited or labeled "unscientific." A documentary exposing flaws in industry practices may quietly disappear from platforms. These aren't conspiracy theories—they're patterns, repeated across decades.

One example that's particularly revealing is the history of dietary fat. For years, fat was vilified based on flawed research, much of it influenced by industry interests. The sugar industry funded studies in the 1960s that downplayed sugar's role in heart disease and shifted the blame to saturated fat. It took decades to undo that damage—decades during which countless people avoided healthy fats, embraced processed "low-fat" products, and experienced a cascade of metabolic dysfunction.

The same is true for environmental toxins. Chemicals like BPA, phthalates, and glyphosate have long been linked to endocrine disruption and chronic illness. Yet efforts to regulate or even warn the public have been slow and fiercely contested—because the industries behind them are powerful and well-protected.

When science is filtered through commercial interests, the truth gets distorted. And for the average person, that distortion can feel like whiplash. One week eggs are healthy, the next they're dangerous. Coffee causes cancer—until it doesn't. Salt is the enemy—until it's not. The confusion isn't accidental. It keeps people overwhelmed, unsure, and reliant on experts to interpret the chaos for them.

And so, over time, we learn to doubt our instincts. We hand over our health decisions to systems that may not have our best interests at heart. We stop asking questions—not because we're lazy or uninformed, but because we've been taught that the answers are too complex for us to understand.

But complexity is not the same as confusion. Much of what supports true health is actually simple, even obvious—when we clear away the noise. Eating food in its natural form. Minimizing toxic exposure. Supporting the body's own intelligence. These truths don't require a degree to understand. What they require is the courage to look beyond what's convenient, and the willingness to rethink what we've been told.

That's where this conversation turns—from the suppression of science to the reclamation of personal responsibility. And that's where we'll continue next.

When we begin to pull back the curtain, what we find is not a lack of information—but an overwhelming flood of filtered, redirected, and sometimes deliberately obscured knowledge. It's not that solutions don't exist. It's that the ones that don't serve the dominant medical-economic model often never see the light of day in the mainstream.

Take, for example, the growing body of evidence around environmental medicine. Researchers and physicians have been pointing to the effects of heavy metals, mold exposure, and chemical sensitivities for decades. Some have published compelling case studies, showing profound improvements when these factors are addressed. Yet most conventional doctors receive little to no training in this area. Why? Because there's no standard pharmaceutical treatment for "detoxing" a home, no blockbuster pill for mold remediation. So these issues remain labeled as fringe, their advocates dismissed as outliers, and patients continue to suffer, misdiagnosed or ignored.

Even within nutrition, the suppression is palpable. Nutritional therapy—rooted in real food, nutrient density, and biochemical individuality—is often brushed aside in favor of standardized dietetics designed around calories, not nourishment. While many clinicians and researchers have long known that micronutrient deficiencies can drive fatigue, mood disorders, and immune dysfunction, these insights rarely get center stage in the health conversation. Why? Because correcting nutrient imbalances isn't profitable. There's no long-term customer in a patient who heals through food.

And yet, this suppression often doesn't come with outright lies. It comes with omission. It's what we're not told that keeps us stuck. We're not told that pharmaceutical trials are frequently funded by the very companies selling the drugs. We're not told that journal editors have spoken out about conflicts of interest that compromise the scientific publishing process. We're not told that many treatments labeled as "evidence-based" have marginal benefits at best when held up to real-world results—and significant risks that are underreported.

But perhaps the most dangerous outcome of all this suppression isn't just misinformation. It's disempowerment. When people sense that they're not being told the whole story—when they hear their doctor dismiss their lived experience, or their concerns get reduced to "anxiety"—they begin to doubt themselves. They start to internalize the idea that maybe they really are imagining things, or worse, that there's no real solution for how they feel.

This creates a dangerous loop. The patient, confused and defeated, turns back to the very system that failed them for another prescription, another specialist, another round of tests. And all the while, the root causes go unaddressed.

Breaking that cycle starts with awareness. We don't need to become conspiracy theorists or reject science altogether. Quite the opposite—we need to reclaim science. True science is not dogma. It's inquiry. It's open, evolving, and inclusive of diverse data. It doesn't silence dissenting voices. It invites them to the table.

For readers of this book, the message is not "don't trust anyone." It's "learn to trust yourself." Your symptoms are not random. Your fatigue is not normal. Your confusion around health is not because you're uneducated—it's because the information has been made confusing on purpose.

Healing starts when we stop handing over all our power and start becoming participants in our own wellness. That doesn't mean you have to do it all alone. It means finding practitioners who listen, who think critically, and who don't treat you like a machine to be fixed, but a person to be understood.

It also means doing the hard, hopeful work of sifting through what's been hidden—and choosing to see with clear eyes. Not everything labeled "alternative" is valid, and not everything "approved" is safe. The truth lives somewhere in between, and often, it's found through curiosity, courage, and critical thinking.

Suppressed science doesn't stay buried forever. It re-emerges through people like you—people who ask better questions, who share what they learn, and who refuse to settle for the version of health that keeps them half-alive.

Let this be the moment you stop being a passive recipient of information and start becoming a seeker of truth. That shift alone is a form of healing. And it's one nobody can censor.

Who Benefits When You Stay Sick?

It's an uncomfortable question, isn't it? Not just *why* so many people are sick today, but *who gains* from it. We're often taught to believe that the health care system is broken—well-meaning, maybe, but overwhelmed and underfunded. But what if it's not broken at all? What if it's functioning exactly as intended?

To begin unpacking that, we need to take a hard look at the incentives. At its core, modern medicine is a business. This isn't a judgment—it's a reality. Hospitals, insurance companies, pharmaceutical giants, and even many research institutions operate within profit-driven frameworks. In this model, a healthy, self-sufficient person isn't particularly valuable. But someone who's chronically unwell, who needs ongoing care, medications, lab work, imaging, and specialist visits? That's recurring revenue. That's a long-term customer.

This is where the system quietly thrives: in managing disease rather than resolving it. It doesn't necessarily require malicious intent. In fact, most individuals within the system—your nurse, your general practitioner, the pharmacist—are compassionate and deeply committed to helping people. But the machinery they operate within is designed to prioritize treatment over root-cause resolution, maintenance over cure, and dependency over autonomy.

Take, for example, the pharmaceutical industry. A massive portion of its revenue comes from what's known as "maintenance medications"—drugs people are expected to take not for days or weeks, but for life. Statins, antidepressants, proton pump inhibitors, blood pressure pills, and diabetes medications are just a few examples. The goal isn't to heal the underlying dysfunction, but to stabilize the symptoms indefinitely.

Now imagine what would happen if those same patients addressed the root causes of their health conditions—perhaps through a combination of nutrition, detoxification, stress regulation, gut healing, and other evidence-informed approaches. Medication need would drop. Doctor visits would decline. Insurance billing would plummet. The entire ecosystem of dependency would begin to erode.

So it's no wonder that approaches aimed at true healing—especially when they involve simple, low-cost, or non-patentable interventions—rarely get serious attention or funding. There's no big financial upside to empowering people to take care of their own health with food, rest, sunlight, and a clean environment. These things don't boost quarterly earnings.

But pharmaceuticals are only part of the picture. The food industry plays a deeply interwoven role here as well. Many of the chronic health conditions plaguing modern society—obesity, diabetes, autoimmune issues, fatigue, mood disorders—have strong dietary links. And yet, processed food companies continue to market ultra-palatable, chemically engineered products that are addictive by design. These foods trigger inflammation, blood sugar dysregulation, gut damage, and more—issues that conveniently require pharmaceutical intervention down the line.

In a darkly ironic twist, you'll often find the very companies that sell junk food funding the campaigns that supposedly raise awareness about chronic illness. A soda manufacturer might sponsor a diabetes walk. A cereal company might back a heart health initiative. The message is clear: "We're all in this together." But we're not. The people making billions off your declining health are not the ones shouldering the consequences.

Let's also not forget the role of media in this equation. Health narratives are shaped not just by science, but by who can afford to promote their message. Pharmaceutical companies are among the largest advertisers on television, online platforms, and even in medical journals. That kind of influence doesn't just buy airtime—it buys silence. It buys favorable framing. It ensures that certain conversations never happen in public.

And so, a person watching the nightly news, reading their favorite wellness blog, or even listening to their doctor may be receiving information that's been shaped—consciously or not—by the needs of the very industries that profit from sickness.

The result of this system isn't just a population grappling with chronic illness—it's a society that begins to accept that being unwell is normal. Feeling tired all the time? Just part of adulthood. Digestive issues? Blame it on stress. Mood swings? Hormones. Brain fog? Aging. We are slowly taught to lower our expectations of health, to silence the signals our body is giving us, and to settle into the idea that there's a pill—or a diagnosis—for everything.

And this conditioning starts early. Many of us grew up watching our parents manage multiple prescriptions. Commercials reinforced the message that health was something to be purchased: antacids for dinner-time bloating, sleep aids for restless nights, energy drinks for chronic fatigue. These weren't temporary fixes for acute issues. They became lifestyle essentials. We didn't just normalize disease—we learned to live around it.

But here's the critical truth: behind every chronic symptom is a signal. The body isn't malfunctioning without cause. It's responding—sometimes desperately—to something in the environment, the diet, the mind, or the internal ecosystem. And often, those causes are modifiable. But getting to the root takes time, awareness, and effort. It also requires stepping outside the dominant system and asking hard questions—about food, medications, chemicals, stress, and even the healthcare model itself.

Unfortunately, doing that often places the burden on the individual. The healthcare system doesn't typically make space for deep investigative conversations. A typical doctor's visit might last 7 to 15 minutes. In that time, there's rarely room to talk about sleep hygiene, the glyphosate in your food, your emotional stress load, or the mold exposure in your home. It's faster, and more "efficient," to offer a diagnosis and a drug. Not because doctors don't care—but because the system doesn't allow them to do more. And yet, this is the very space where healing begins—when someone pauses long enough to ask, "What's really going on in my body?" When we stop outsourcing our health completely and start rebuilding our connection to it. It's in this shift, from passive patient to active participant, that we start to reclaim control.

This isn't about rejecting medicine. There's a vital place for it, especially in emergencies, surgeries, and acute care. But what we're addressing here is chronic, lifestyle-driven illness—the kind that now makes up the overwhelming majority of doctor visits. The kind that the system, as it stands, is not designed to prevent or reverse.

So when you ask, "Who benefits when I stay sick?" the answer is complex. It includes pharmaceutical shareholders. Food conglomerates. Insurance companies. Even parts of the wellness industry that sell false hope through endless supplements or detox fads. But the cost isn't just monetary—it's physical, emotional, generational.

You pay with your energy, your presence, your clarity. Your relationships suffer. Your work, your passions, your ability to show up for life get filtered through a fog of discomfort or dysfunction that you've been told is simply part of life.

But there's another path—one where health isn't something you chase, but something you reclaim. One where you learn to read your body's cues instead of silencing them. Where food becomes fuel, rest becomes sacred, and clarity replaces confusion.

That path isn't funded by billion-dollar campaigns. It won't be suggested in a 30-second commercial. It doesn't come in a quick fix. But it's real, and it's within reach. And the moment you begin to ask the question—*Who benefits when I stay sick?*—you begin to shift the power dynamic. You begin to remember that your health is yours.

And that, perhaps, is the most revolutionary thing of all.

PART II — The Reset Protocol

There comes a moment, after the shock of realization and the flood of frustration, when something shifts. You stop looking outward for permission and start listening inward for direction. This is the turning point—the moment you decide to do something different. Not because it's trendy or easy, but because your body is asking for it. Your symptoms aren't random. They're signals. And now, you're ready to respond.

This part of the book is where we stop circling the problem and start moving toward the solution. But not in the form of a magic pill or a miracle diet. What you'll find here is a grounded, evidence-aligned roadmap for recalibrating your system. It's not about overhauling your life in a week. It's about making the invisible visible again—seeing where toxins have crept in, where resilience has worn thin, and where healing has been waiting for space to happen.

The Reset Protocol isn't a detox gimmick. It's a return to the body's natural rhythm. We'll explore what's really in your food, water, and environment—and how to reduce your daily toxic load in realistic, sustainable ways. You'll learn how gut health impacts everything from your brain to your immune system. We'll talk about the role of chronic inflammation, how it shows up, and what helps bring it down. This isn't theoretical—it's practical, doable, and designed to work with your life, not against it.

Most importantly, this section is built around clarity and empowerment. You don't need to know everything. You don't need to get it perfect. You just need to begin. One choice at a time. One habit at a time. One day at a time.

This is where the reset begins—not just for your body, but for the relationship you have with it.

Let's get started.

Detoxing the Hidden Toxins

What's Lurking in Your Food, Water, and Home

We tend to trust the environments we live in. The food we eat, the water we drink, the air we breathe—it's easy to assume they're safe. After all, aren't there regulatory agencies, safety standards, and experts tasked with protecting us? But that trust has quietly been eroded, and most people don't even realize it. We've grown used to toxins, contaminants, and hidden chemicals woven into our daily lives. So much so, that we no longer question what "normal" really means.

Walk through any grocery store and look at the shelves. The ingredients in the average household pantry are a chemistry set. Artificial dyes, preservatives, industrial oils, emulsifiers, and synthetic sweeteners are not exceptions—they're the norm. And they're not harmless fillers. Many of these substances have been linked in studies to chronic inflammation, gut disruption, and even neurobehavioral issues. Yet they're allowed. And worse, they're not even labeled in ways the average person can understand or evaluate.

Take seed oils, for instance. Marketed as "heart healthy" alternatives to saturated fats, oils like canola, soybean, and corn oil are industrial byproducts extracted using high heat and chemical solvents. When consumed regularly, they contribute to oxidative stress and systemic inflammation. You wouldn't drink machine lubricant, but these oils aren't far off from that in terms of how they affect the body over time.

The situation with water isn't much better. Municipal tap water often contains trace pharmaceuticals, pesticide runoff, heavy metals, and chemical byproducts like chlorine and chloramine. In some areas, fluoride is still added to the water supply—not the natural kind found in soil and mineral springs, but a synthetic industrial version, often derived from fertilizer production. While fluoride is marketed as a dental benefit, the long-term health effects of chronic exposure, especially in children, are still debated among researchers. More concerning is that most people have no idea what's actually in their tap. Even when water meets the official "safe" limits, it doesn't mean it's optimal—or even healthy over decades of use.

Our homes, too, have quietly become reservoirs of low-grade toxicity. Consider your cleaning products, your shower curtain, your mattress, your air fresheners. Many of these everyday items off-gas volatile organic compounds (VOCs), endocrine-disrupting chemicals like phthalates, or flame retardants that persist in dust. We inhale them, absorb them through our skin, and accumulate them slowly—while rarely noticing any immediate symptoms. But over time, the exposure adds up. Fatigue, hormonal imbalances, poor sleep, brain fog—these can all stem from chronic environmental toxin overload.

Then there's the food packaging. Plastics that leach bisphenol A (BPA) or its cousin BPS. Cans lined with endocrine disruptors. Nonstick pans releasing PFOAs into your meals. Even so-called "healthy" foods often come in packaging that compromises the very integrity of what's inside.

It's easy to feel overwhelmed. The toxins are everywhere. But the purpose of this chapter isn't to scare you—it's to make you aware. You can't change what you don't see. Once you recognize what's happening, you can begin to shift. And the shifts don't need to be drastic or expensive to be effective. The goal is not to create a perfectly pure life (which is nearly impossible), but a lower-toxin, more intentional one.

Let's begin in the kitchen. Swapping out harmful ingredients isn't about perfection—it's about progress. Start by shifting away from ultra-processed foods. These often contain dozens of synthetic additives, stabilizers, and preservatives that your body doesn't recognize. When you can, choose whole foods—single-ingredient items with no label or a very short one. Trade industrial oils like canola or soybean for olive oil, avocado oil, or ghee. Not only are these more stable under heat, but they also support better hormonal and cellular health.

Pay close attention to how your food is stored and cooked. Plastic containers, especially when heated, can leach hormone-disrupting chemicals into your meals. Opt for glass, stainless steel, or silicone instead. Nonstick pans, especially older ones, may still contain PFOA or other persistent compounds that have been linked to serious health effects. Replacing them with cast iron, ceramic, or stainless steel can significantly reduce your exposure.

Water filtration is one of the most powerful and overlooked investments you can make in your health. Even a basic carbon filter pitcher can reduce chlorine, some pesticides, and pharmaceutical residues. For deeper filtration—especially if your area has known heavy metals or fluoridation—a reverse osmosis system or a gravity-fed multi-stage filter may be worth considering. These don't just improve the taste of your water; they help lessen the long-term toxic burden on your kidneys, liver, and brain.

Now think about your air. Indoor air pollution is often worse than outdoor, especially in modern homes with poor ventilation. Scented candles, synthetic air fresheners, and conventional cleaning sprays might make your house "smell clean," but they're often saturating your air with VOCs, phthalates, and other toxins that disrupt your nervous and endocrine systems. Instead, look for fragrance-free or essential oil–based alternatives, or even simple homemade solutions using vinegar and baking soda. Adding plants like peace lilies or snake plants can also help filter the air, though they're a complement—not a substitute—for good ventilation and cleaning up the source.

The bathroom is another hidden source of chemical exposure. Many personal care products contain a cocktail of ingredients that may interfere with your hormones over time—things like parabens, formaldehyde-releasing preservatives, and synthetic fragrances. The skin is highly absorptive, so what you put on your body matters. It's not about throwing everything out at once. Start with the items you use daily and apply to large areas—like lotion, deodorant, and body wash—and slowly transition to cleaner versions.

Even your laundry routine can be a hidden problem. Conventional detergents and fabric softeners often contain harsh chemicals and artificial scents that linger on your clothes and bed sheets. Since you wear and sleep in them, you're getting hours of exposure every day. Switching to fragrance-free or naturally derived options can dramatically reduce your toxic load with minimal effort.

The key here isn't to fear your home—it's to reclaim it. Toxins have become so normalized that we often don't notice them until our bodies begin to break down. But your body has an incredible ability to heal and regulate, especially when you remove what's constantly disrupting it.

This isn't about selling expensive solutions or becoming obsessive. It's about understanding the silent burdens many people live with unknowingly. Once you reduce that burden—bit by bit—you may notice your energy improving, your mind becoming clearer, your immune system becoming more resilient. These aren't magical promises. They're physiological realities your body has always been capable of—if given the chance.

You deserve to live in a home that supports your well-being. You deserve food that nourishes, not harms. And you deserve to know the truth about what you're really being exposed to every single day. Awareness is the first step, but action is what creates change.

What's next is learning how to remove toxins more actively and restore the systems that have been working overtime to protect you. Because once you know what's lurking, you're no longer powerless. You're in charge—and that changes everything.

How to Remove Toxins Naturally

After becoming aware of the hidden toxins that accumulate in our daily lives—from food to water to household products—the next logical question becomes: how do we actually get them out of our bodies?

Fortunately, your body isn't defenseless. You are not a passive victim of toxicity; you're equipped with a finely tuned detoxification system—your liver, kidneys, skin, lymphatic system, and gut all work together to neutralize and eliminate harmful substances. The problem is, in our modern world, these systems are often overwhelmed. They're doing their job nonstop, without enough support, rest, or resources. Natural detox isn't about trendy cleanses or quick-fix teas. It's about giving your body the tools, space, and time it needs to do what it was designed to do.

It all starts with reducing the ongoing input of toxins. You can't out-detox a toxic lifestyle. If you're constantly adding in harmful substances—through what you eat, breathe, or apply to your skin—your body never gets the break it needs to catch up. That's why step one of any effective detox is subtraction. Subtract the inflammatory foods. Subtract the toxic cleaners. Subtract the synthetic chemicals in your skincare. As those inputs are removed, the body begins to shift from survival mode into restoration.

Hydration is the next cornerstone. Water is more than just a thirst quencher—it's a detoxifier's best friend. Every cell in your body requires adequate water to function properly. Your kidneys flush out water-soluble toxins through urine. Your lymphatic system, which carries waste away from tissues, depends on hydration to flow efficiently. Your skin relies on hydration for proper sweating. But not all water is created equal. Clean, filtered water—free from heavy metals and chlorine—is the ideal foundation. Adding a pinch of mineral-rich salt or a squeeze of lemon to your water can also help replenish electrolytes and gently stimulate detox pathways.

Next comes nourishment. Your liver—the main organ of detox—requires specific nutrients to process toxins safely. B vitamins, glutathione, sulfur compounds from foods like garlic and onions, antioxidants from leafy greens, and amino acids from clean proteins all support its work. Fiber, especially from vegetables and seeds, acts like a broom in your gut, binding to toxins and helping escort them out through the stool. Without enough fiber, toxins processed by the liver can actually be reabsorbed back into circulation, making you feel worse over time.

Movement is a surprisingly vital piece of natural detox. When you move your body—whether through walking, stretching, or gentle strength training—you activate circulation, stimulate the lymphatic system, and encourage your body to release waste through breath, sweat, and improved digestion. Unlike your blood, which is pumped by your heart, the lymphatic system requires physical motion to flow. Sedentary lifestyles create stagnation—not just in energy, but in waste clearance. Even 10 minutes of movement in the morning can activate these systems and prime your body for a healthier day.

Sweating is one of the body's most underrated detox tools. Through sweat, the body can eliminate heavy metals, BPA, phthalates, and other fat-soluble toxins. This is one reason sauna therapy, especially infrared saunas, has grown in popularity among functional medicine practitioners. But you don't need fancy tools. A brisk walk, a hot bath with Epsom salts, or time outdoors on a warm day can help your body do what it naturally wants to do—offload.

While most people understand detox as a purely physical process, what's often overlooked is the emotional and energetic residue we carry—experiences, traumas, beliefs, and stressors that don't just impact our minds but leave physiological imprints. Chronic stress, for example, disrupts your hormonal balance, impairs digestion, and lowers your body's detox capacity. You can be eating all the right foods and moving your body daily, but if you're emotionally flooded, your system is still under strain.

This is where practices like breathwork, meditation, journaling, or simply spending time in nature can have a profound effect. They activate the parasympathetic nervous system—your body's rest-and-digest state—which in turn enhances digestion, liver function, and lymphatic flow. Creating moments of calm each day isn't just about reducing stress; it's about creating biological conditions for healing. Emotional hygiene is just as essential as physical hygiene when it comes to detoxifying your life.

The skin, as your body's largest organ, is also a crucial player in detoxification. It acts as a secondary elimination channel, especially when the liver and kidneys are overburdened. Skin eruptions, rashes, or excessive oil production can often be signals of internal congestion. Support your skin's ability to detox by allowing it to breathe—literally. Opt for natural skincare products free of parabens, synthetic fragrances, and petrochemicals. Let your skin sweat when it needs to. And occasionally, allow yourself to go without cosmetics to reduce the absorption of additional chemicals.

Your gut, too, plays a pivotal role. It's not just where nutrients are absorbed—it's where many toxins are either expelled or recirculated. When your gut barrier is compromised (a condition often referred to as "leaky gut"), substances that should stay in the digestive tract can leak into the bloodstream, triggering systemic inflammation. A healthy gut means strong mucosal integrity, robust microbial diversity, and regular elimination. Eating fermented foods, rotating your produce, and avoiding unnecessary antibiotics are all practical ways to support the gut's detox function.

And then there's sleep—arguably the most powerful, free, and underutilized detox tool of all. While you sleep, your brain activates its glymphatic system, a fluid-based process that flushes out waste products, including beta-amyloid plaques linked to cognitive decline. Sleep also gives your liver and kidneys time to perform their tasks uninterrupted. That "brain fog" so many people report isn't just mental fatigue—it's often a signal that your internal waste systems didn't get the rest or resources they needed the night before.

It's important to understand that real detoxification is not a quick fix or a one-time cleanse. It's a daily rhythm, a slow and steady recalibration. There is no need for extreme deprivation, juice-only diets, or expensive supplements marketed as miracle detoxifiers. What your body needs is consistency. That means prioritizing clean food, safe water, conscious movement, stress reduction, and rest—all on a regular basis.

You don't need to do it all at once. Start by focusing on the inputs: what you eat, drink, breathe, and absorb through your skin. Then begin layering in the outputs: supporting elimination pathways through hydration, bowel regularity, sweating, movement, and sleep. Notice how your body responds—how your energy changes, how your skin clears, how your mind feels less cluttered. These are signs of real progress.

When you remove what weighs the body down, it remembers how to thrive. It doesn't need to be forced—it simply needs the interference to stop. Detox is ultimately a return to your body's original intelligence. It's not about punishing your body into compliance. It's about clearing the path so your health can finally move forward, unhindered.

And when you feel that shift—not just physically, but mentally and emotionally—you begin to understand what real vitality feels like. It's not perfection. It's clarity, strength, and resilience coming back into focus. And it starts with choosing, day after day, to support your body's natural ability to heal.

Daily Habits That Keep You Toxic (And What to Replace Them With)

Many of the habits we carry into our everyday lives feel harmless—normal, even. We trust our routines. We buy what's sold to us. We follow advice that seems conventional. But what if some of those daily choices are quietly filling our bodies with stress, chemicals, and inflammation? What if the "normal" habits we've inherited are not just unhelpful, but actively contributing to the fatigue, bloating, brain fog, and chronic symptoms so many people now accept as part of life?

The truth is, many modern habits are inherently toxic. Not toxic in a dramatic, catastrophic way—but in a slow-drip, accumulative way that wears down the body's natural defenses over time. It's not the one fast-food meal or the one late night that breaks the system. It's the repetition of these habits, day after day, layered with other stressors and exposures, that eventually overloads the body's ability to detox, reset, and heal.

Start with what you put in your body every morning. For many people, the day begins with a cup of coffee—on an empty stomach. The caffeine jolts the adrenal glands, sending a false stress signal before any real nourishment has arrived. Paired with a breakfast of processed carbs or nothing at all, this routine sets off a blood sugar rollercoaster that can impact mood, focus, and hormones for the rest of the day. You may not feel the crash immediately, but it shows up later—maybe as irritability, sugar cravings, or that mid-afternoon slump.

Then there's your environment. You get ready with products you trust: shampoo, deodorant, lotion. But flip the bottle around and the ingredients list reads more like a chemistry worksheet. Synthetic fragrances, parabens, phthalates—many of these are known endocrine disruptors. Day after day, they absorb through the skin, bypass the liver's first-pass filtration, and begin to accumulate in tissues. Because these chemicals are present in low doses, they fly under the radar of regulation. But that doesn't mean they're harmless.

Move into the kitchen. How often do we microwave leftovers in plastic containers? Or store food in them for days at a time? Plastics can leach hormone-mimicking compounds into our meals, especially when heated. Even "BPA-free" plastics aren't necessarily safe—many use replacement chemicals that may be just as problematic. Similarly, non-stick cookware, while convenient, often relies on coatings that release toxins when scratched or overheated.

And consider hydration. Most people don't drink enough water—and when they do, it's often from bottled sources that have been sitting in plastic for weeks or months, potentially exposed to heat during transportation. Tap water, though a better option in some cases, can still carry contaminants like chlorine, fluoride, heavy metals, and pharmaceutical residues. These may be present in small quantities, but again, the body notices what you repeat. What you consume consistently becomes part of your internal environment.

Let's also talk about movement—or lack thereof. A sedentary lifestyle is often framed as a productivity requirement, especially in the digital age. We sit for work, sit for leisure, sit while we eat. But movement isn't just about burning calories. It's about circulation, lymphatic flow, digestion, and detoxification. Without physical movement, the lymph system—which is responsible for clearing waste—becomes stagnant. You might feel puffy, sluggish, or mentally foggy, not because of what you ate or how much you slept, but because your body hasn't had the chance to circulate and release.

Then there are the screens. Most of us are surrounded by them—from the phone we scroll before bed to the computer that commands our daylight hours. Screens are not just visual distractions; they emit blue light that suppresses melatonin, disrupts sleep, and interferes with the body's repair cycles. Over time, overstimulation from constant digital engagement can raise cortisol levels, dysregulate circadian rhythms, and contribute to emotional exhaustion.

Once you begin to see these patterns for what they are—not random but repetitive, not neutral but cumulative—it becomes easier to shift. And the shift doesn't need to be extreme. It's not about perfection. It's about awareness, and then gently choosing what serves your body rather than burdens it.

Start by revisiting your morning routine. Instead of reaching for coffee before anything else, consider waking up with a glass of mineral-rich water—ideally with a pinch of unrefined sea salt and a squeeze of lemon. This simple act rehydrates the body after sleep, supports the adrenals, and signals your system that nourishment, not stress, is the first order of the day.

If you do drink coffee, try pairing it with a small meal containing healthy fat and protein to stabilize blood sugar and reduce the spike–crash cycle.

In your bathroom, small swaps make a big difference over time. You don't need to throw out everything overnight. As you run out of each product, replace it with something simpler—cleaner. Look for personal care items made with plant-based ingredients, free of artificial fragrances and preservatives. Your skin is not a barrier; it's a gateway. What you put on it matters.

In the kitchen, prioritize food storage and heating methods that don't leach harmful compounds. Glass containers are a reliable option, both for storage and reheating. If that's not accessible right away, at least avoid heating plastic in the microwave. When it comes to cookware, stainless steel, cast iron, or ceramic-coated pans are safer bets. These may seem like minor decisions, but over time they reduce your body's exposure to hormone disruptors and heavy metals.

Water is foundational, so give it the attention it deserves. Investing in a quality water filter can dramatically lower your exposure to contaminants. There's no need for an expensive or elaborate system—just one that removes common toxins like chlorine, lead, and volatile organic compounds. And instead of plastic bottles, aim for a glass or stainless-steel bottle you can refill throughout the day. It's not just better for you—it's better for the planet too.

Now let's talk about movement. You don't need a gym membership or a fitness tracker to support your detox pathways. What your body craves is consistency. A daily walk. Gentle stretching. Breathwork. Lymphatic flow is stimulated by movement, even small movements. Rebounding on a mini-trampoline for a few minutes a day, for instance, is a simple but powerful way to help your body clear waste. What matters is that you interrupt long periods of stillness with moments of intentional motion.

And for your nervous system, which is perhaps the most overlooked player in the detox equation, consider how you wind down at night. Swap the last hour of scrolling for a ritual that helps you disengage and reset. That might be reading, journaling, light stretching, or simply dimming the lights and letting the mind rest. Melatonin, your sleep hormone, needs darkness and calm to be released. Without it, the body loses its rhythm and healing slows.

The truth is, toxic habits often stick not because we love them, but because they're familiar. We've been conditioned to follow convenience, not consciousness. But your body has always been speaking to you. Through headaches, through fatigue, through bloating and breakouts—it's been asking for relief. When you start removing the quiet poisons of everyday life, you begin to hear its voice more clearly. And when you listen, healing becomes much less complicated.

What we often call "detox" isn't something extreme or rare. It's something your body is doing all the time. The real question is whether your daily habits are supporting that process—or silently blocking it. By replacing toxic routines with more natural, aligned choices, you give your system the space it needs to do what it already knows how to do: restore, renew, and return to balance.

The shift may be gradual. But the benefits—clearer thinking, deeper sleep, stable energy, better digestion—are hard to ignore. And they're not the result of chasing another product or protocol. They come from removing what doesn't belong. That's the real medicine. Not more, but less. Not adding, but subtracting the things that no longer serve you. And that, in itself, is a profound act of healing.

Gut, Brain, and Inflammation Reset

The Gut–Mind–Body Connection

For decades, the body was treated like a collection of isolated parts. Your brain was a thing "up there," your gut a thing "down there," and whatever connected the two was largely ignored. But science—and more importantly, lived experience—is painting a different picture. One that recognizes that your gut is not just about digestion, and your mind is not just about thoughts. They are part of the same continuous, communicating system. And when one suffers, the other does too.

You've probably heard the gut referred to as your "second brain." That's not just a catchy phrase. It's a reflection of something real: your gut has its own nervous system, known as the enteric nervous system, and it's home to over 100 million nerve cells. This isn't a backup system—it's a dynamic command center that constantly sends messages to your brain, influencing mood, memory, focus, and even behavior. And the reverse is also true. What's happening in your mind—stress, anxiety, emotional patterns— deeply affects what's going on in your gut.

Have you ever felt your stomach twist before a big decision? Or lost your appetite during a period of grief? Or had unexplained digestive issues during stressful life phases? These aren't coincidences. They're evidence of the gut–mind connection in action. And if your gut is inflamed, out of balance, or compromised in any way, it can disrupt your mental clarity and emotional stability without you even realizing it.

What often gets overlooked is how this connection influences your entire system. The gut is where around 70% of your immune system lives. It's where neurotransmitters like serotonin—often associated with mood and well-being—are primarily produced. It's also where inflammation often begins, quietly, before it manifests as something more noticeable: joint pain, fatigue, skin issues, mental fog, or persistent low mood.

The trouble is, most people don't link their bloating or irregularity with their anxiety. Or their skin issues with their bowel movements. Or their depression with what they ate for dinner last night. We've been conditioned to compartmentalize symptoms and to treat them in isolation. But the human body doesn't work that way. Everything is connected. The gut influences the mind. The mind affects the gut. And both together shape how your body functions every day.

Modern life, unfortunately, is not kind to this connection. Processed foods disrupt the microbial balance in your gut. Pesticides damage the intestinal lining. Chronic stress tightens the digestive system and compromises nutrient absorption. And antibiotics—while sometimes necessary—can wipe out the beneficial bacteria that help you stay emotionally and physically resilient.

It's important to understand that healing your gut isn't just about digestion—it's about recalibrating your entire internal communication network. A gut that's in balance sends calm, steady signals to the brain. It tells the body, "We're safe. We're nourished. We're okay." But a gut in distress sends signals of alarm, confusion, or depletion. And those signals don't just stay in your belly—they influence how you think, how you feel, how you show up in the world.

This is why symptoms like brain fog, mood swings, and chronic fatigue often don't get better with therapy alone. Or with supplements alone. Or with medications alone. They require a deeper look into what's happening in the body—specifically, the gut—and how it may be impacting your emotional and cognitive state.

Healing the gut isn't a trendy health goal—it's a foundational process for reclaiming your full vitality. When the gut is cared for, the mind feels clearer. When the mind is less reactive, the body rests and restores more easily. It's a loop, not a ladder. And the entry point is different for everyone.

Now we'll explore what it really takes to rebuild that gut–mind–body harmony—starting with how your microbiome shapes your inner world far more than you've probably been told.

The gut microbiome—an ecosystem of trillions of bacteria, viruses, and fungi living in your digestive tract—plays a massive role in how you feel, think, and function. It's not just a passive community; it's an active player in your emotional and physical reality. Some strains of gut bacteria are linked with calmness and emotional balance. Others are associated with inflammation, irritability, and even depression. When that ecosystem is out of balance—a state called dysbiosis—everything else begins to drift off course.

This is why someone can be eating "healthy" by conventional standards, yet still feel bloated, anxious, or emotionally reactive. It's not just what you eat—it's what your body can digest, absorb, and harmonize with. A diet high in processed foods, sugar, artificial additives, and low in fiber can gradually starve beneficial bacteria and feed the more disruptive ones. Over time, the messaging system between your gut and brain becomes distorted. The result is not always immediate digestive distress. Sometimes it's mental. Sometimes it's emotional. Sometimes it's subtle—just enough to make you feel like you're always "off," but not enough to know exactly why.

Repairing this connection begins by removing the daily stressors that weaken the gut lining and throw the microbiome into disarray. These aren't just food-related; emotional and environmental toxins are part of the picture too. Chronic stress, for example, can thin the lining of the intestines, leading to what's often referred to as "leaky gut." When that barrier becomes permeable, undigested food particles, toxins, and microbes can slip into the bloodstream and trigger inflammation—both physical and psychological.

You might feel this as irritability, scattered thoughts, tension in the body, or a sense of being emotionally fragile. The mind may race. Sleep may become shallow or restless. Your nervous system begins to live in a hyper-alert state, even if you're not aware of it. And from that state, true healing becomes much harder.

The way forward is not just about probiotics or another supplement stack. It's about creating a daily environment—inside and out—that supports safety, nourishment, and rhythm. The gut thrives on consistency. When meals are eaten mindfully, when the body is given a chance to rest, and when stress is gently processed rather than suppressed, the microbiome can begin to stabilize.

Movement helps too. Not strenuous exercise necessarily, but natural movement—walking, stretching, breathing deeply. These actions send signals to the gut that the body is not in danger, that it can digest, absorb, and repair. The body is wired to heal, but only when it's not in survival mode.

Equally important is emotional hygiene—tending to your inner life with honesty and care. Suppressed emotions, unresolved grief, or long-held tension don't just stay in the mind. They register in the gut. They alter the tone of your nervous system. They affect which bacteria flourish and which fade away. When you begin to express, release, and reconnect with your inner world, your body responds too. Digestion improves. Sleep deepens. Thoughts become clearer.

It's a powerful feedback loop—one that doesn't require perfection, just presence. Listening to your body, learning its signals, and responding with patience and respect begins to rebuild a foundation that no pill can replicate. Healing the gut–mind–body system isn't about chasing symptoms. It's about restoring harmony to a system that has long been overstimulated and undernourished.

So if you've been living with chronic brain fog, mood swings, unexplained fatigue, or that feeling of never quite being "right" in your body—consider this: maybe it's not all in your head. Maybe it's in your gut. And maybe, by nourishing that forgotten center, you unlock a clarity and energy that's been missing for far too long. This is the power of reconnection. And it begins with awareness.

Chronic Inflammation: The Root of Modern Illness

You can't see it in the mirror, and you might not even feel it in any obvious way, but chronic inflammation could be quietly shaping your entire health story. Unlike the kind of inflammation you get from a cut or a sore throat—where redness, heat, and swelling alert you to a problem—chronic inflammation simmers beneath the surface. It's slow. It's subtle. And it's often dismissed as unrelated to the symptoms we live with daily.

But this invisible process plays a central role in nearly every major health crisis of our time. From autoimmune conditions and cardiovascular disease to depression, fatigue, and even Alzheimer's, chronic inflammation is the common thread woven into the background. It isn't just a side effect. It's often the root.

So how did we get here? How did a biological process designed to protect us become the very thing that breaks us down?

Inflammation itself is not the enemy. In fact, it's essential. When your body is exposed to injury or infection, inflammation is the first responder. It sends immune cells to the area, clears out damaged tissue, and kickstarts healing. That's acute inflammation—short-lived, controlled, and purposeful.

The problem begins when the body doesn't turn off the alarm. Instead of resolving the response, it keeps sounding it, day after day, year after year. The immune system remains activated, and instead of repairing, it begins to overreact. Healthy cells and tissues start to suffer. The body, in its attempt to protect, becomes its own threat.

This chronic inflammatory state often begins silently, sparked by factors so common in modern life that we've stopped questioning them. Diets loaded with processed food, sugar, and industrial oils feed inflammation. Sedentary lifestyles leave the body stagnant and under-oxygenated. Poor sleep disrupts the body's natural repair cycles. Long-term exposure to environmental toxins—found in everything from cleaning products to plastic packaging—adds fuel to the fire. And then there's stress, perhaps the most underestimated of all, subtly triggering inflammatory responses through hormonal shifts that were never designed to be long-term.

What makes chronic inflammation so insidious is its ability to shape-shift. It rarely shows up as a single, easily identified problem. Instead, it manifests as a collection of vague symptoms: joint pain, low energy, brain fog, bloating, skin issues, headaches, mood swings. Often, these complaints are treated as isolated issues or brushed aside as normal signs of aging or stress. But behind them, inflammation may be quietly at work.

Doctors may prescribe a cream, a pill, or a new diagnosis, but rarely is the deeper question asked: *Why is the body inflamed in the first place?*

This question is vital, because when inflammation is left unchecked, the body begins to adapt in unhealthy ways. It might suppress immune function in one area while ramping it up elsewhere, creating a confused and chaotic internal environment. Over time, this imbalance increases the risk of chronic illness—not just in the body, but in the mind as well. Depression, anxiety, and cognitive decline have all been linked to inflammatory markers in the bloodstream.

And yet, for something so deeply connected to modern disease, chronic inflammation still doesn't get the attention it deserves. Mainstream health conversations tend to focus on surface-level solutions: treating a diagnosis instead of the process that led there. It's like trying to patch up leaks in a dam without addressing the rising pressure behind it.

To truly heal, we have to start upstream. That means recognizing inflammation for what it is: a signal. Not an enemy to silence, but a messenger asking us to listen. When the body is inflamed, it's not just malfunctioning—it's trying to communicate.

Now that we've explored how inflammation begins and why it's so widespread, let's turn our attention to the next crucial piece: how to calm it. Because the good news is, even long-standing inflammation can be reversed. But the process doesn't begin with a supplement or a prescription. It begins with reclaiming the basics. And that's where we'll go next.

Calming chronic inflammation isn't about adding more noise to your life. It's about quieting the storm that's been brewing beneath the surface—sometimes for years. And to do that, we start with the foundations your body was always designed to rely on: nourishment, movement, rest, and rhythm.

Let's begin with food. It's not just fuel; it's information. Every bite you take sends a message to your body—either one that amplifies inflammation or one that soothes it. Ultra-processed foods, refined sugars, and inflammatory oils like soybean and canola whisper the wrong message day in and day out. They confuse your cells, exhaust your immune system, and disrupt the gut lining, allowing harmful compounds to leak into the bloodstream and keep the immune response on high alert.

Contrast that with a meal built from whole, colorful vegetables, omega-3-rich fats, healing herbs, and clean proteins. This kind of nourishment tells the body it's safe. It supports tissue repair, gut healing, and hormonal balance. It helps the immune system return to a state of calm vigilance rather than constant overdrive. The goal isn't perfection—it's awareness. Most people don't realize that what they call "normal eating" is often keeping their bodies in a state of silent alarm.

Then there's movement—not punishment in the form of intense workouts, but movement as medicine. Gentle walking, stretching, strength training, and time spent outdoors all improve circulation, oxygen delivery, and lymphatic flow. The lymphatic system is crucial here—it's the body's waste disposal system, and unlike the heart, it has no pump. It depends on your movement to function. Without it, toxins linger, and inflammation persists. Equally vital is sleep. Chronic inflammation doesn't stand a chance against true, consistent rest. But too many people live in a constant state of sleep debt, mistaking five or six broken hours for enough. During deep sleep, the body clears out cellular waste, balances blood sugar, and reduces cortisol, the stress hormone. But when rest is shallow or erratic, the body stays in defense mode. That might look like increased pain, irritability, or the inability to lose weight—yet few connect those dots back to the lack of restorative sleep.

Speaking of cortisol, chronic stress is one of the most powerful and underestimated drivers of inflammation. The body doesn't distinguish between the threat of a predator and the anxiety of unread emails, constant notifications, or financial pressure. It responds the same way: by releasing stress hormones that, over time, compromise immune function, damage the gut lining, and feed systemic inflammation.

This is why lifestyle isn't separate from health—it is health. What you think, how you breathe, the pace at which you live, all of it shapes your biochemistry.

You don't need to overhaul your life in a single week. But you do need to start listening. What are the messages your body has been trying to send you for years? Maybe it's the headaches you've normalized. The digestive issues

66

you've medicated. The brain fog you laugh off. Maybe it's fatigue that no amount of caffeine seems to solve.

All of these are invitations to go deeper. To stop chasing surface solutions and start addressing the internal imbalance that fuels them.

The body wants to heal. It's hardwired for it. But it needs the right environment. Removing inflammatory triggers is one half of the equation. The other half is restoring the conditions that allow repair: safety, nourishment, movement, and stillness.

As we move forward in this journey, keep this truth close: chronic inflammation is not a life sentence. It's a red flag. And when you respond to it with intention and awareness, you'll find that symptoms begin to shift—not because you suppressed them, but because you listened.

Healing is not about silencing your body. It's about finally hearing it—and giving it what it's been asking for all along.

Heal the Gut, Heal the Body

You've probably heard the phrase "health begins in the gut," but few people truly understand what that means—until their body starts to fall apart in ways that conventional medicine can't explain or fix. The truth is, the gut is far more than just a place where food is digested. It's a command center for the immune system, a regulator of mood and brain function, a frontline of defense, and a critical player in inflammation, detoxification, and hormone balance. When it's compromised, everything else is compromised too.

Most people walk around with some level of gut dysfunction and don't even know it. Bloating after meals, frequent fatigue, skin flare-ups, anxiety, recurring infections, joint pain—these are not separate issues. They are the scattered signals of a system trying to communicate that something is off at its core.

And the core, more often than not, is the gut.

This isn't a fringe idea. The gut microbiome—a vast ecosystem of bacteria, viruses, fungi, and other microbes—has been the subject of intense scientific interest over the last decade. We now know that the balance of these microorganisms determines how effectively your body absorbs nutrients, how well your immune system responds to threats, and even how your brain functions. But here's the problem: modern life is not built to support a healthy gut. It's built to destroy it.

From the foods we eat to the pace we live, most daily habits are unknowingly hostile to gut health. Refined sugar, seed oils, artificial additives, alcohol, antibiotics, pesticides, and even chronic stress all erode the delicate balance of the microbiome. They strip away beneficial bacteria and encourage the overgrowth of harmful strains. Over time, the protective lining of the gut—the mucosal barrier—becomes inflamed and damaged. Tiny gaps begin to form in the gut wall, allowing undigested food particles, pathogens, and toxins to "leak" into the bloodstream. This is what's commonly referred to as leaky gut, and it's not rare—it's rampant.

The immune system, always alert for danger, recognizes these intruders and launches an attack. That attack becomes chronic when the leaks don't stop. And that's where the cascade begins: inflammation, food sensitivities, autoimmune conditions, hormonal imbalances, mental health issues. The body becomes a battleground.

The conventional approach is to chase the symptoms—treat the rash, suppress the anxiety, medicate the fatigue—but the root remains unaddressed. Healing has to start from within, and the gut is ground zero.

But here's the empowering truth: just as the gut can be damaged over time, it can also be healed. It responds, sometimes remarkably quickly, to the right conditions. This isn't about following a rigid diet or buying expensive supplements. It's about rebuilding trust with your body. Giving it the nourishment, rest, and care it's been deprived of for too long.

Healing the gut doesn't begin with doing more—it begins with removing what's been harming it.

That's where most people get stuck. They want to know what to add without letting go of what's breaking them down. But as long as the gut remains inflamed and overburdened, even the most nutrient-dense foods or powerful probiotics won't land the way they're meant to. It's like pouring clean water into a dirty glass—you still get murky results.

The first steps of true gut healing are about subtraction. Removing the common irritants, the inflammatory triggers, the hidden disruptors. And not just in food, but in lifestyle—because what you digest isn't limited to meals. Your nervous system digests your environment, your relationships, your pace of life.

That's where we'll pick up next: how to begin creating the internal and external conditions that allow the gut to repair, re-seal, and re-balance—so the rest of the body can finally follow.

So, how do you actually begin the process of healing your gut?

It starts with simplifying. The gut is not asking for complexity—it's asking for relief. For many people, that means taking a hard look at the foods they've accepted as "normal" but are silently inflammatory. Processed grains, refined sugars, seed oils, and conventional dairy may not spark an immediate reaction, but over time, they contribute to a steady drip of irritation that keeps the gut lining raw and the microbiome off balance.

Replacing those with whole, nutrient-dense, unprocessed foods makes a dramatic difference. Bone broth, for example, is rich in collagen and glutamine—two compounds that directly support the rebuilding of the intestinal wall. Fermented foods like sauerkraut and kefir can help reintroduce beneficial bacteria, while prebiotic foods like garlic, onions, and asparagus provide the fuel those good microbes need to thrive.

But food is only one piece of the puzzle.

The gut and nervous system are deeply connected. In fact, the gut is sometimes referred to as the "second brain" because it produces neurotransmitters like serotonin, dopamine, and GABA. That connection goes both ways—meaning that if your life is filled with chronic stress, no amount of kale or kombucha will fully fix what's broken. When the body is stuck in fight-or-flight mode, digestion slows, inflammation rises, and gut permeability worsens.

That's why gut healing also means stress healing.

It means slowing down. Creating moments of stillness. Learning how to breathe fully again. It may sound too simple, but rest is medicine for the gut. When the parasympathetic nervous system is activated—what we call the "rest and digest" state—the body finally has permission to do what it's designed to do: repair.

Movement matters, too. Not as punishment, but as support. Gentle walking after meals, stretching, yoga, or mindful exercise can help stimulate digestion and circulation, which are crucial for nutrient delivery and detoxification. You're not just healing the gut—you're restoring flow through the whole system.

Then there's the role of sleep. Deep, restorative sleep is when the gut does much of its repair work. Poor sleep disrupts microbial balance and increases inflammation, creating a vicious cycle that's hard to break without intervention. For many people, prioritizing sleep—cutting screens at night, establishing a wind-down ritual, staying consistent with bedtime—is one of the most potent forms of gut medicine available.

And finally, patience.

This is perhaps the most overlooked part of healing. We live in a culture addicted to quick fixes, instant results, and 30-day transformations. But your body doesn't operate on deadlines. It heals in seasons, in layers, and in ways that don't always follow a straight line. Some days you'll feel better, other days you won't. That's not failure—it's recalibration.

What matters is that you stay in relationship with your body through the process. Listening. Adjusting. Trusting. The more you shift from controlling the body to cooperating with it, the more profound the results will be.

Because gut healing is not just a physical process—it's an emotional and energetic one, too. The gut holds so much more than food. It holds anxiety, grief, tension, and unprocessed life. As it begins to heal, don't be surprised if old emotions rise to the surface. That's part of the detox. That's part of the reset.

So, "heal the gut, heal the body" isn't a slogan—it's a biological and emotional truth. When the gut is whole, the body feels safe again. Inflammation settles. Energy returns. Hormones balance. Mood lifts. And most importantly, you begin to feel like *you* again—not the version of you that's been surviving, but the version that's finally thriving.

The path to health doesn't start with chasing symptoms. It starts with rebuilding the foundation. And the gut is where that foundation lives. Treat it with respect, give it what it needs, and your whole body will thank you—quietly, steadily, and over time, completely.

Energy, Hormones & Metabolic Repair

Why You're Tired No Matter How Much You Sleep

You drag yourself out of bed in the morning even though you got a full night's sleep. You yawn through meetings, feel your energy flatline mid-afternoon, and rely on caffeine or sugar just to stay upright. You might even hear yourself say, "I'm always tired," without really knowing why.

And you're not alone.

Fatigue is one of the most common, yet least understood complaints in modern health. Millions of people feel exhausted every day despite "doing all the right things." They sleep 7 to 9 hours a night, they try to eat well, maybe even exercise—yet the tiredness lingers like a fog that never lifts. So what's going on?

First, it's important to realize that sleep quantity and sleep quality are not the same thing. You can be in bed for eight hours and still wake up feeling like you haven't rested at all. That's because your body isn't just counting hours—it's counting the depth of your repair. And when your body is inflamed, stressed, overburdened by toxins, or hormonally out of balance, the quality of your sleep suffers even if you're getting enough of it on paper. One major culprit is **hidden inflammation**. Chronic low-grade inflammation can interfere with your sleep architecture—those deep, restorative stages of sleep that allow your brain and body to detoxify and reset. You might not feel sick, but your body is working overtime behind the scenes trying to put out internal fires. This constant demand for repair drains your reserves and keeps you stuck in a state of underlying fatigue.

Then there's the role of **blood sugar**. Most people don't realize how much unstable blood sugar impacts energy. If your meals are loaded with processed carbohydrates or sugars—even the so-called "healthy" ones—they can cause spikes and crashes throughout the day. These crashes don't just affect mood or hunger; they also affect cortisol and adrenaline, both of which play key roles in energy regulation. Over time, this roller coaster leads to deeper fatigue, brain fog, and the feeling that your energy simply isn't reliable anymore.

But perhaps the most overlooked factor of all is **mitochondrial dysfunction**. Your mitochondria are the microscopic energy factories inside your cells. They take nutrients and oxygen and convert them into the energy your body needs to function. When they're compromised—whether by environmental toxins, poor diet, lack of movement, or chronic stress—your body can no longer produce energy efficiently. You're running on fumes, and no amount of sleep can fill that tank if the engine itself is broken. So, while it's easy to blame tiredness on a "busy lifestyle" or getting older, the real issue is usually deeper. Your body isn't lazy. It's trying to tell you something.

This is where many people get stuck. They start adding supplements, trying new sleep hacks, or doubling down on willpower to get through the day. But they never stop to ask the real question: *Why isn't my body restoring itself when I sleep?*

Because true rest doesn't happen just because the lights are off.

Your body can only enter deep, restorative states if it feels safe—physically, chemically, and emotionally. If you're going to bed wired from stress, if your liver is overburdened by toxins, if your gut is inflamed, or your hormones are imbalanced, your body spends the night defending itself instead of repairing itself.

We'll dive deeper into those specific systems shortly. But first, let's unpack how chronic stress rewires your internal rhythm—making you tired and wired at the same time—and why many people are unknowingly living in survival mode even while they sleep.

Living in a state of chronic stress has become so normalized that many people no longer even recognize it as stress. They just call it "life." But when your nervous system is constantly activated—rushing from one task to the next, mentally juggling responsibilities, worrying about the future, or even just being exposed to overstimulating environments—your body doesn't get the message that it's safe to downshift.

This state is known as sympathetic dominance, or "fight-or-flight" mode. And the more time you spend in it, the harder it becomes to access true rest. Even when you sleep, your system is on alert, scanning for danger. This isn't conscious; it's physiological. Your heart rate doesn't fully drop, your breath stays shallow, your muscles stay slightly tense, and your brain can't fully drop into the deep waves necessary for cellular repair. So you wake up just as tired—sometimes even more so.

What adds to the confusion is that many people feel wired at night but exhausted during the day. This is a key sign of a disrupted circadian rhythm, often caused by artificial lighting, late-night screen exposure, skipped meals, or caffeine consumed too late in the day. Your internal clock runs on cues—light, food timing, movement. When those cues are off, your melatonin and cortisol rhythms flip, leading to sluggish mornings and restless nights.

Sleep is no longer the reset it's meant to be.

Hormones also play a critical role in this picture, especially for women. Fluctuations in estrogen and progesterone can affect not only mood and metabolism but also energy and sleep cycles. If your body is under chronic stress, it prioritizes cortisol production over sex hormones, leading to imbalances that further disrupt your ability to rest and repair. This is why so many women in perimenopause or menopause report increased insomnia and fatigue—even when their routines haven't changed.

Then there's the overlooked link between gut health and sleep. The gut produces a large portion of the body's serotonin, a neurotransmitter that is a precursor to melatonin—the sleep hormone. When the gut is inflamed, overrun by dysbiosis, or undernourished, this serotonin-melatonin conversion gets impaired. You may fall asleep, but the depth and quality of that sleep suffer. And over time, so does your energy.

So what's the way out?

The first step is to shift the question from "How can I force myself to sleep better?" to "What's preventing my body from accessing its natural rhythm of rest and repair?"

It's about clearing the noise—reducing the inflammation, supporting your gut, nourishing your mitochondria, and restoring safety to your nervous system. This doesn't happen overnight. But it starts with awareness: understanding that your body isn't broken, it's overwhelmed. And the tiredness you feel is not weakness—it's feedback.

Begin to look at energy not as a motivational issue, but as a biological signal. Start eating in a way that stabilizes your blood sugar—regular meals that include healthy fats, proteins, and fiber to avoid the highs and lows that wear out your adrenals. Focus on gentle movement that calms your nervous system, like walking or stretching, especially in the morning light to reset your circadian clock. Carve out screen-free time in the evening. Not for perfection, but for rhythm.

And perhaps most importantly, begin to rebuild trust with your body. That means listening. Slowing down when you're exhausted instead of pushing through. Prioritizing deep rest—not just sleep, but mental and emotional exhale. Creating spaces where your body can stop bracing and start restoring.

Because when your body feels safe, energy returns.

True vitality isn't something you chase—it's something that returns when the obstacles are removed. And your tiredness is not the enemy. It's the beginning of a conversation. One that, when answered with compassion and curiosity, can lead you back to the kind of rest that truly restores.

Resetting Hormones Naturally

Most people think of hormones as something that only becomes relevant during puberty, pregnancy, or menopause. But in reality, your hormones are working every minute of every day to regulate your energy, mood, metabolism, sleep, immune function, libido, and so much more. When they're balanced, you feel grounded and steady. When they're not, it can feel like your body is fighting against you—emotionally and physically.

Yet in modern life, hormonal imbalances are not the exception anymore. They've quietly become the norm.

It's not just women, and it's not just aging. More and more men are facing plummeting testosterone levels at younger ages. Women are seeing symptoms of estrogen dominance, adrenal fatigue, and thyroid dysregulation even in their 20s and 30s. What's even more concerning is how often these symptoms are normalized—chalked up to being "just tired," "just anxious," or "just getting older." Fatigue, brain fog, irritability, stubborn weight gain, low sex drive, restless sleep—these aren't personality traits. They're red flags from your endocrine system.

The hormonal chaos so many people face isn't random. It's a response to constant disruption.

Think about what your hormones are trying to do. They're messengers. They coordinate systems. They maintain homeostasis. But for them to do that, the environment has to be relatively stable. That includes your internal environment—blood sugar levels, gut health, stress chemistry—and your external one: sleep cycles, toxic exposure, light patterns, and food quality.

When you eat processed food, get poor sleep, absorb synthetic chemicals, and live under chronic stress, your hormones don't just "take a hit"—they adapt. But that adaptation often leads to dysfunction. Your body downregulates certain hormones and overproduces others to compensate, creating an internal feedback loop that eventually feels like burnout, mood swings, or metabolic resistance.

Cortisol is one of the main culprits in this loop. Known as the stress hormone, cortisol is necessary in the right amounts—it helps you wake up in the morning, respond to danger, and regulate inflammation. But when cortisol is chronically elevated from too much stress (emotional, physical, or environmental), it begins to suppress other key hormones like thyroid hormones, sex hormones, and melatonin.

This is why people under constant stress often report symptoms like weight gain, insomnia, and cold hands and feet. It's not just stress—it's the hormonal shifts stress sets in motion.

Another core piece of the hormonal puzzle is insulin. This hormone is responsible for moving sugar out of your blood and into your cells for energy. But when you're constantly snacking, living on refined carbs, or skipping meals only to binge later, your insulin has to work overtime. Over time, this leads to insulin resistance—a state where your cells stop responding properly to insulin, causing your body to produce even more of it. The result? Blood sugar crashes, energy dips, weight gain around the midsection, and even hormonal cross-talk that disrupts estrogen and testosterone levels.

This is where many people get stuck. They try to address each symptom in isolation—taking melatonin for sleep, drinking more coffee for energy, or using medication to force hormone levels back into range. But true balance doesn't come from forcing the body. It comes from creating the right environment so your hormones can naturally recalibrate.

That's what a natural hormone reset is about.

And it begins not with restriction, but with restoration—restoring rhythm, nourishment, and safety in the body so that it no longer has to compensate in dysfunctional ways.

Restoration begins with rhythm. Hormones work on cycles—circadian rhythms that govern sleep and energy, monthly cycles that shape reproductive hormones, and even seasonal shifts that influence metabolism and mood. When these rhythms are disrupted by artificial light, erratic eating patterns, or high-stress environments, hormone production becomes disoriented.

To help your body remember its natural rhythm, one of the most powerful tools is light. Morning sunlight on your skin and eyes (without sunglasses or windows in between) signals your brain to regulate cortisol, serotonin, and melatonin production. This one habit alone can improve energy during the day and deepen your sleep at night, setting the stage for more balanced hormonal cascades.

Eating in rhythm matters too. Constant grazing or eating late at night doesn't allow insulin, cortisol, or digestive hormones the space to stabilize. Introducing predictable mealtimes, with enough time between meals for insulin to fall and digestive rest to occur, creates hormonal spaciousness. Your body thrives when it knows what to expect.

Sleep is another pillar. Deep sleep is when your body produces growth hormone, regulates melatonin, and resets cortisol patterns. Even one night of disrupted sleep can throw your hormone levels off for days. This is why good sleep hygiene—like avoiding blue light in the evening, keeping your room cool and dark, and having a consistent bedtime—isn't just a nice-to-have. It's a foundational hormonal strategy.

But rhythm alone isn't enough. The body also needs nourishment—not just calories, but the micronutrients and building blocks required for hormone synthesis.

Cholesterol, for example, has been villainized for years, but it's actually the raw material from which your body makes sex hormones like estrogen, progesterone, and testosterone. Without enough healthy fats in the diet—like those from egg yolks, avocados, olive oil, and pasture-raised meats—your body doesn't have the resources it needs to function hormonally. This is especially important for people coming off long periods of restrictive dieting or chronic low-fat eating.

Magnesium, zinc, selenium, and B vitamins all play crucial roles in hormone production and detoxification. A deficiency in any one of these can slow down hormone metabolism, leading to imbalances that feel like PMS, low libido, hair thinning, or thyroid issues. Whole foods, not supplements, should be your first source of these nutrients. Leafy greens, seeds, wild-caught fish, liver, and quality proteins support hormonal harmony at the root level.

Then there's the need for safety. When your nervous system feels under threat—whether from emotional stress, trauma, toxic relationships, or physical overexertion—your body deprioritizes reproductive and thyroid hormone production. In that state, survival always comes first. Healing requires sending your body the signal that it's safe again.

This is where nervous system regulation and emotional support come in. Breathwork, nature walks, creative expression, time spent with safe and uplifting people—these are not extras. They are medicine for your hormones. They downregulate chronic cortisol elevation and allow your parasympathetic nervous system (your "rest and digest" mode) to dominate again, making space for restoration.

It's also essential to support your body's ability to clear out excess hormones. The liver and gut play key roles here. If your liver is overburdened by alcohol, processed food, or environmental toxins, it can't properly metabolize and deactivate hormones. Similarly, if your gut microbiome is imbalanced or constipated, used hormones can be reabsorbed into your system, perpetuating estrogen dominance and other disruptions. A fiber-rich, whole-foods diet that supports liver detox and regular elimination is one of the most effective ways to keep hormonal signals clean and clear.

None of this is about perfection. It's about consistency and reconnection. Your body is always seeking balance—it just needs you to remove the blocks and provide the support. When you begin to eat in rhythm, sleep in darkness, nourish your cells, and live in a way that reinforces safety instead of stress, your hormones start to respond. Not overnight, but steadily.

And when that balance returns, everything shifts. Energy stabilizes. Moods level out. The weight you've been fighting against begins to release. Your cycle regulates. Your sleep deepens. And most importantly, you feel like yourself again—not someone broken or unpredictable, but someone in sync with your own biology.

That's the power of a natural hormone reset. It's not a detox or a diet—it's a return. A return to the way your body was always meant to work, before it was thrown off by a world that forgot how to live in harmony with it. Now, you remember. And that changes everything.

Metabolic Myths That Keep You Stuck

For years, people have been told that metabolism is simply about calories in and calories out—as if your body were a basic equation on a chalkboard. Eat less, move more. That's the prescription repeated like gospel across magazines, clinics, and diet apps. And yet, millions follow this formula and still feel exhausted, frustrated, and stuck.

Why? Because the story we've been given about metabolism is incomplete—and in many cases, flat-out wrong. Metabolism isn't just about how quickly you burn calories. It's a reflection of your body's overall cellular health, hormonal balance, nervous system function, nutrient availability, and more. It's not a singular switch you can flip on with a treadmill and turn off with a slice of cake. It's a complex and dynamic orchestra, and when one section is out of tune, everything is affected.

One of the most damaging myths is the idea that a "slow metabolism" is a life sentence—that some people are simply cursed with bad genes and destined to struggle. But most so-called slow metabolisms aren't genetic at all. They're adaptive. They slow down in response to stress, nutrient deficiencies, chronic dieting, inflammation, and toxic overload. Your body isn't broken; it's protecting you. When it doesn't feel safe, it conserves energy.

That means the very things people are told to do to "speed up" their metabolism—like cutting calories drastically or overexercising—can actually have the opposite effect. Prolonged restriction triggers your body to lower thyroid hormone output, increase cortisol, and reduce reproductive function, all in an effort to preserve life. It's a survival response, not a failure. But it becomes a trap when misunderstood.

Another popular myth is that exercise alone is the key to a fast metabolism. While movement is essential, it's not the silver bullet many hope for. Overtraining, especially in a depleted state, can place added stress on the body and actually suppress metabolic function. What's often more effective is strategic, moderate movement—like walking, resistance training, or gentle interval work—combined with recovery, nourishment, and nervous system support. The body thrives on balance, not punishment.

Then there's the belief that aging automatically slows metabolism. It's true that hormonal shifts and changes in muscle mass can influence energy needs over time, but much of the metabolic decline blamed on age is actually the result of accumulated stress, inflammation, and poor lifestyle habits—not age itself. When you support your body properly, metabolism can remain strong and responsive well into later life.

We also can't ignore the myth that metabolism is just about weight. In reality, it touches every aspect of your health—your energy levels, mental clarity, digestion, sleep, mood, immune function, and even how quickly you recover from illness. When metabolism is suppressed, everything feels harder. And when it's supported, everything feels lighter, clearer, more stable.

To reset your metabolism, you have to move beyond willpower and into wisdom. You need to unlearn the cultural conditioning that equates health with restriction and thinness with virtue. You need to understand that metabolism is not a number on a chart—it's a sign of how well your body feels supported, nourished, and safe.

The good news is, your metabolism is always willing to respond. It's adaptable. It's forgiving. But first, you have to stop fighting it. You have to stop treating your body like a machine that needs to be hacked or punished. And you have to start treating it like the intelligent, self-regulating system it is.

Rebuilding your metabolism begins with rebuilding safety in your body. This might sound abstract, but it's deeply physiological. Your body is constantly scanning your environment—internal and external—for signals of safety or threat. If it perceives chronic stress, starvation, inflammation, or toxic exposure, it downregulates functions that aren't immediately necessary for survival. Metabolism is one of the first to take the hit.

Let's take a closer look at how these signals play out.

If you're constantly under-eating—skipping meals, cutting carbs, or living off caffeine—your body doesn't interpret that as you "being good." It registers scarcity. And when your brain senses scarcity, it adjusts hormone output accordingly. Thyroid hormones drop. Sex hormones decline. Cortisol rises. Blood sugar becomes more erratic. All of this puts your metabolism in defense mode, not optimization mode.

If you're living in fight-or-flight—waking up with anxiety, rushing through your day, eating on the go, reacting to every ping from your phone—your nervous system is in sympathetic dominance. That alone can suppress digestion, disrupt hormone rhythms, impair sleep, and signal to your body that this isn't a good time to expend energy. Your body doesn't prioritize fat-burning when it thinks it's running from a threat. It holds on. It conserves.

And if you're flooded with environmental toxins—pesticides in your food, plastics in your water, synthetic fragrances in your home—your liver and detox systems are constantly working overtime. This overload can impair your body's ability to convert hormones, break down nutrients, and eliminate waste efficiently—all of which feed back into metabolic health. A sluggish detox system often translates to a sluggish metabolism.

So what do you do?

You start by sending your body the opposite signals. You create safety instead of stress. You feed it consistently with real, nutrient-dense foods. You balance meals to keep blood sugar stable. You rest. You walk. You breathe deeply. You start your mornings with grounding rather than stimulation. You reduce inputs that overwhelm and replace them with rhythms that restore. This isn't about extremes—it's about regulation.

You also begin to reframe your relationship with food. Instead of asking, "How little can I eat and still get through the day?" you ask, "How can I nourish myself in a way that supports healing and vitality?" That shift alone can begin to reset patterns that have kept you stuck. Food becomes fuel, not the enemy. And you stop micromanaging your calories and start listening to your body's cues.

Equally important is releasing the guilt and shame that often come with "failed" attempts at health. If you've followed mainstream advice for years and ended up more tired, more inflamed, and more confused—that's not your fault. You weren't given the whole story. And in many cases, you were given advice that worked against your body rather than with it.

Healing begins when you let go of punishment and lean into partnership. You stop trying to "fix" your metabolism like it's broken and start asking what it's trying to tell you. You recognize that symptoms are signals, not defects. They're your body's way of communicating its needs. And when you listen—really listen—you'll be guided toward what supports true repair. What you'll likely find is that restoring metabolism isn't about doing more—it's about doing what matters. It's about consistency, not intensity. It's about simplicity, not complication. And it's about honoring the deep intelligence of your body instead of overriding it.

Your metabolism wants to support you. It wants to give you energy, clarity, strength, and resilience. But it can't do that if it's constantly in defense mode. When you shift the inputs—when you stop sending stress and start sending safety—you'll begin to feel the shift. Your energy will return. Your brain will clear. Your body will respond.

And the myths? They'll fall away. Because you'll no longer need them.

You'll be living proof that healing is possible when you stop fighting your biology and start working with it. That's the true reset. Not a trick. Not a trend. A return to your body's original design—where wellness isn't forced, it's restored.

The 7-Day Reset Plan

Preparing Your Body and Mind

Before any real transformation can begin, there must be a preparation phase — not just physically, but mentally and emotionally. This is the step most people skip. They go straight to action: the detox, the meal plan, the supplements. But when the body and mind aren't prepared, even the best protocols can feel like a fight. You're not just asking your system to do something new; you're asking it to let go of patterns, defenses, and beliefs that have been deeply wired over time.

True healing isn't just about what you do — it's also about how you enter the process. Are you rushing in from a place of fear or frustration? Are you hoping for a quick fix because you feel broken or betrayed by your own body? Or are you stepping in with curiosity, compassion, and the willingness to show up for yourself in a new way?

Preparing your body means starting gently. Many people carry years — or decades — of inflammation, toxicity, and stress. Jumping into aggressive detox or major dietary overhauls without foundational support can backfire. Your organs may not be ready to process and eliminate the backlog. This doesn't mean you're fragile. It means you're wise to create stability first.

That starts with nourishment. Not just with food, but with rest, rhythm, and hydration. Before removing or changing anything, it's powerful to simply focus on adding: more minerals, more water, more quality sleep, more moments of stillness. These are not just soft lifestyle upgrades — they are biological requirements for healing. When the nervous system begins to calm, when digestion starts to work more efficiently, when your cells are better hydrated, the entire body becomes more responsive.

Your nervous system is the gatekeeper of healing. If you're constantly wired, tense, or overstimulated, your body stays in survival mode. And healing does not happen in survival mode. It happens in safety. So part of preparation is learning how to send your system the signal that it's okay to let go. This might be through breathwork, time in nature, journaling, or even just slowing down your mornings. These small shifts tell your body: you're not in danger. You can heal now.

Equally important is preparing your mind. If your mental landscape is filled with doubt, overwhelm, or unrealistic expectations, you will sabotage yourself before you even begin. You've likely been conditioned to believe that health is a battle — that your body is broken, that symptoms are enemies, that more effort equals better results. These ideas are not neutral. They create tension and resistance. They make you fight yourself.

So take a moment before diving into anything new to examine what you actually believe about your body. Do you believe it's capable of healing? Do you believe that you can trust your intuition, or are you waiting for someone else to give you permission? Are you holding onto past failures as proof that this won't work? These thoughts matter. They shape your choices, your consistency, your resilience when things get uncomfortable — because at some point, they will.

This phase is not about perfection. It's about presence. It's about choosing to become the kind of person who is available for healing, not just the kind who is chasing it. That means embracing a mindset of readiness, not urgency. You're not rushing to fix yourself. You're laying the foundation for a new relationship with your body.

Now we'll explore how to practically support this preparation with specific daily rhythms and mindset anchors — the kind that don't just make healing possible, but sustainable. Because preparation is not a pause before the work begins — it is the work. And if you honor it, your results won't just be faster. They'll be deeper, truer, and longer-lasting.

Let's begin with rhythm. Your body thrives on rhythm — not rigid routines, but a natural, repeatable flow. The more erratic your sleep, meals, and movement patterns are, the harder it becomes for your system to stabilize. Preparation, then, is partly about reclaiming rhythm. Start waking up and going to bed at the same time. Begin your day with intention — not by grabbing your phone or reacting to emails, but by giving your body a moment of stillness, hydration, and breath.

Drinking a glass of clean water first thing in the morning isn't just hydration — it's a ritual of return. You're signaling to your cells that you are here, present, and choosing to begin again. Add a pinch of sea salt or a squeeze of lemon if you like — something to tell your nervous system: "We are not in chaos today."

Then move your body. Not because it burns calories or tones muscles, but because movement wakes up your circulation, your lymph, your digestion. It helps clear stagnation — physical, emotional, energetic. Even five minutes of stretching or a short walk can shift your state. The point isn't performance. It's presence. You're not preparing for a marathon. You're preparing for clarity.

On a mental level, one of the most powerful tools you have is awareness. Start noticing what triggers your stress response. Is it a specific task, a food, a relationship dynamic, or even just your thoughts? Awareness doesn't require you to fix everything all at once. It just asks you to look without judgment. The moment you become aware of a pattern, you're no longer fully controlled by it.

This is also a time to simplify. Your nervous system is more likely to reset in a space that's not overloaded. Try decluttering one small area of your environment — not to be productive, but to signal that you're making space for something new. Clear space often mirrors a clear internal state.

From here, begin engaging your senses. Play calming music, use essential oils you enjoy, sit in the sunlight for five minutes. These aren't just nice extras — they are cues. They speak to your limbic system, which governs emotion, memory, and survival. When you engage your senses in gentle, nurturing ways, you send the message that the world is safe — and so are you.

Mentally, this is the moment to reconnect with your why. Not the surface-level reasons like losing weight or looking better — but the real why. Maybe it's wanting to feel present with your children. Maybe it's not being afraid of food anymore. Maybe it's freedom from fatigue, or finally trusting your body again after years of frustration. Write it down. Revisit it. This is your anchor.

You may find yourself slipping into old stories during this preparation phase — the belief that you don't have time, that you've failed before, that you'll never figure it out. These are echoes from a mindset of survival. You're not in that space anymore. The work you're doing now — simply showing up, simplifying, listening — is how you begin to rebuild trust with your body.

And that trust is what changes everything. When your body feels safe, it releases. When your mind feels seen, it softens. And when your habits are rooted in intention rather than punishment or fear, they start to feel effortless — not because they're easy, but because they are aligned.

Preparing your body and mind is not just a one-time phase. It becomes a lens through which you engage with your entire healing journey. You're not trying to arrive at some perfect version of yourself. You're becoming someone who supports yourself in real time — with flexibility, honesty, and care.

In the next stages of this book, we'll walk together into the more active parts of the reset process — the detoxification, the rebuilding, the re-patterning. But everything starts here. With rhythm. With awareness. With a willingness to slow down and listen. Because healing isn't something you chase. It's something you allow. And when you prepare well, you don't just change your habits — you change your relationship with your own life. That's where true reset begins.

The Daily Reset Ritual (What to Eat, Think, and Do)

We tend to think that change requires big, dramatic action. A detox, a cleanse, a diet overhaul. But the truth is, the body responds more to what you do consistently than what you do intensely. A reset isn't a single event — it's a quiet rhythm you return to each day. And when that rhythm is built with care, everything changes.

The Daily Reset Ritual is not a rigid checklist. It's a living practice — something you craft to support your body, your mind, and your nervous system in real-time. It's less about discipline and more about alignment. And when you build your day around a few simple, intentional anchors, your body stops fighting and starts healing.

It starts the moment you wake up. Not with your phone. Not with a to-do list. But with presence. Before the world rushes in, give yourself two minutes of stillness. Sit up in bed, place your feet on the floor, and breathe. Feel your body. Remind yourself that you're here. That you're safe. That you are choosing to reset — not to fix yourself, but to support yourself.

Then hydrate. After hours without water, your body is thirsty — not just for hydration, but for flow. A large glass of filtered water, maybe with a pinch of real salt or a squeeze of lemon, tells your system it's time to wake up. It's a signal. And your body responds to signals far more than it responds to rules.

Movement comes next. Not punishment, not exhaustion — just movement. Five minutes of stretching, a walk around the block, gentle breathwork. It's about energy circulation. Moving your body in the morning supports lymphatic drainage, mental clarity, and metabolic readiness. And more importantly, it grounds you. You feel your feet. You come back into your body.

Now let's talk about food. The point of a daily reset is not to eat "perfectly." It's to eat in a way that stabilizes you. That supports your energy rather than spiking and crashing it. Breakfast should be simple, balanced, and real. Something with fat, fiber, and protein — maybe eggs with sautéed greens, chia pudding with almond butter, or a smoothie with clean protein and avocado. No sugar rush. No caffeine on an empty stomach. Just nourishment.

What you eat is only part of it. How you eat matters just as much. Sit down. Breathe before you begin. Chew slowly. Put your fork down between bites.

This is how digestion actually begins — not in your stomach, but in your nervous system. If your body doesn't feel safe, it doesn't absorb. The ritual is presence, not perfection.

Mid-morning is where many people crash — not because they're broken, but because their blood sugar was never stable to begin with. If that's you, this is your cue to slow down and nourish again. A handful of raw nuts, a boiled egg, some cut veggies with hummus. Not because you "should" — but because your body is asking for steady fuel.

And here's where we introduce the second pillar of the reset: your thoughts. Throughout the day, the way you think becomes just as influential as the way you eat. What do you say to yourself? Are you spinning in judgment, comparison, or anxiety? Are you rushing, pushing, proving? The daily reset ritual means pausing — for just 30 seconds — to check in.

Where is your mind? Where is your breath?

The point of these check-ins isn't to control your mind but to reclaim your awareness. Most people spend their day reacting — to noise, to pressure, to endless pings and demands. But your nervous system isn't built for that. It's wired for rhythm, for slowness, for recovery. Just one breath can remind your body that it's not in danger. That you can pause. That you are not your pace.

This is why, during a reset, your midday habits matter just as much as your morning ones. If your day turns into a blur, your body does too. Digestion slows. Focus scatters. Mood drops. So around midday, carve out space to eat with intention again. Choose food that leaves you steady and clear — nothing fried, nothing artificial, nothing that makes you feel heavy or jittery. A grounding bowl, a warm soup, some clean protein with leafy greens. You're not chasing a rulebook. You're listening.

And while your body eats, let your mind rest. Step away from your screen. Chew slowly. Let your body shift into "rest and digest" mode. That alone can change everything. When you're calm, your body absorbs more. It heals faster. It communicates better. What's simple becomes powerful.

As the day progresses, energy naturally shifts. You're not supposed to feel like a machine. There's a soft dip in the afternoon — and rather than pushing through it with caffeine, you can use that window for gentle realignment. Stretch your legs. Step outside. Breathe deeply. This isn't wasted time; it's what allows your system to regulate instead of burn out.

And then comes the evening — the most overlooked part of the daily ritual. By nightfall, most people are overstimulated and undernourished, exhausted but wired. They scroll instead of connect. They eat out of habit, not hunger. They collapse into bed without actually winding down. This is where the reset truly deepens — not in what you remove, but in what you replace.

Start small. Dim the lights. Shut down screens. Give your body cues that it's safe to soften. A warm herbal tea, a magnesium soak, or five quiet minutes with a book can be more healing than any supplement. Your body doesn't need more data; it needs space to process the day and restore balance.

Dinner should be your lightest, most digestible meal. It's not a punishment — it's support. Your body wants to clean, repair, detox overnight. If it's burdened with a late heavy meal, it can't do that. But if you give it simple nourishment — maybe a bowl of broth with vegetables, or a baked sweet potato with a handful of greens — it responds with clarity and deep rest.

And that brings us to the final pillar: sleep. Not just quantity, but quality. Restorative sleep begins hours before your head hits the pillow. It's shaped by every choice you made during the day — your hydration, your blood sugar, your movement, your mindset. If your days are chaotic, your nights will be too.

So let sleep be sacred. Not something you earn, but something you protect. Create a sleep window. Honor it. Let your room be cool, dark, quiet. Let your thoughts unwind, your breath slow, your body sink into stillness. This is when your nervous system reboots, your hormones regulate, your cells regenerate. It is, quite literally, your most powerful reset.

In the end, the Daily Reset Ritual is not about doing everything perfectly. It's about choosing to come back to yourself — again and again. It's about replacing noise with clarity, urgency with rhythm, depletion with nourishment. You don't need to fix your body. You need to remember how to support it.

And when you do, healing doesn't feel like a fight anymore. It feels like a homecoming.

What to Expect and How to Stay Consistent

No matter how prepared you feel, beginning a full-body reset is never just about what's on your plate or in your supplement drawer. It's about what comes up — emotionally, physically, and even spiritually — when you begin disrupting the patterns that have silently shaped your life.

At first, the shift might feel subtle. You're drinking more water. Eating cleaner. Making time for breath, stillness, or mindful routines. These early steps can feel empowering — like you're finally taking control of something that once felt out of reach. But right alongside the empowerment, a quieter tension often appears: doubt, impatience, even resistance. And this is where many people start to question if they're doing it "right."

Here's the truth: it's normal for your body and mind to push back at first. When you remove the everyday toxins — physical or emotional — the system scrambles to recalibrate. This isn't failure. This is healing in motion. Detox symptoms may surface, like mild fatigue, skin breakouts, brain fog, or emotional ups and downs. The body isn't breaking down — it's releasing. You're loosening years of accumulation. Don't rush this. Don't fear it. Give your body the respect it deserves for taking on the work.

Consistency during this time becomes your anchor. Not perfection — consistency. It's not about "never slipping." It's about choosing to return, even after a setback. A missed reset meal or a stressful day doesn't undo your healing. The deeper win is in how quickly and gently you return to alignment.

What helps most during this early stretch is understanding your why. Why are you here? Why did you decide to reclaim your health? It's easy to get distracted by short-term discomfort if you lose sight of your long-term vision. Write it down. Speak it aloud. Feel it in your bones. Whether it's being fully present for your kids, waking up with energy, or living pain-free, that vision is your lifeline when motivation wavers.

And motivation will waver. This is another truth many don't talk about. You won't wake up every day excited to meditate, stretch, or cook clean meals. You might get bored. You might feel lonely. You might look around and see others still living the way you used to — fast, loud, numb — and feel tempted to go back. This is part of the path. Growth isn't glamorous. It's gritty. But the peace that follows is unlike anything you've ever known.

It's also important to prepare for how others may respond to your reset. When you start making different choices, some people might not understand. They might tease you. Or feel judged by your change, even if you say nothing. This isn't about them. It's about what your transformation mirrors back to them. Let that go. Stay kind, stay clear, and stay grounded in your choice. You don't need permission to heal.

Some days will feel seamless. Other days, it will take everything you have to stay on course. That's when rituals matter most — the small, stabilizing anchors you return to even when life feels chaotic. Maybe it's starting your morning with lemon water, stretching for five minutes, or sitting quietly with your breath before bed. These aren't just habits. They are lifelines.

As your reset deepens, you may notice an emotional unveiling that catches you off guard. This is a natural, often overlooked part of healing. The body stores unresolved emotions — grief, anger, disappointment — in tissues, especially when they've been ignored or numbed for years. As the toxins clear, so do some of these emotional layers. You might find yourself crying for no apparent reason, feeling irritable, or even experiencing moments of deep stillness you haven't felt in decades. Don't pathologize this. Let it move. Let it speak.

Staying consistent means welcoming these shifts instead of trying to control or suppress them. Remember, the body is not just detoxing what you've eaten — it's detoxing what you've endured. And sometimes what you've believed. Long-held beliefs like "I'm just a tired person," or "I always get sick," or "health is for other people" begin to unravel as you nourish yourself more deeply. This is powerful, and it can feel disorienting. If your identity has been wrapped around fatigue or struggle, living from a new state — energy, clarity, vibrancy — might even feel foreign.

This is why consistency must be anchored in self-compassion. You are not becoming someone new; you are returning to someone you've always been underneath the noise. There's nothing to prove. No one to impress. Each choice you make to stay present with your body, to nourish rather than punish, is a declaration: I am worth taking care of. This isn't about chasing an aesthetic or a quick fix. This is about sustainability — a health that holds you for life.

One of the most practical tools for staying consistent is tracking how you feel, not just what you do. Instead of obsessing over perfect meals or checking boxes, begin to journal or reflect on what's shifting in your energy, your digestion, your mood, your sleep. The real transformation often hides in these subtle changes. Maybe your skin is clearer. Maybe your mind feels less scattered. Maybe you're more patient with your kids. These are wins that matter. Celebrate them. Reinforce them.

Another overlooked part of consistency is forgiveness. You will have off days. You may eat something that throws your system off. You might skip your rituals for a week. What matters is that you don't let these slips harden into shame. Shame disconnects. It makes you forget your power. Instead, use those moments as signals — not failures, but feedback. What's out of alignment? What do you need to return to yourself? Healing isn't linear. It's cyclical. And that cycle includes grace.

Lastly, remember that consistency is a rhythm, not a race. It's not about rigid discipline or hyper-productivity. It's about weaving your reset into the fabric of your life in a way that supports you. For some, that might mean batch cooking on Sundays. For others, it might mean saying no to one obligation a week to make space for rest. Find your rhythm. Let it be yours. When you personalize your path, it becomes less about willpower and more about resonance. You're not forcing yourself — you're following your truth. And that's what this reset is really about: not just detoxing your body, but rebuilding trust. Trust in your body's intelligence. Trust in your ability to change. Trust that healing is possible, even if the world told you otherwise. You were never broken — just overloaded. And now, you're remembering how to listen. How to support. How to stay.

This is the work that lasts. Not because it's flashy or dramatic, but because it's rooted. And anything rooted has the power to grow. Keep choosing that. Keep coming home to yourself. One consistent, loving step at a time.

PART III — Sustained Transformation

You've come a long way. If you're reading this section, it means you've not only opened your eyes to the hidden patterns that have been undermining your health — you've also begun to take action. You've peeled back the layers, questioned old narratives, and perhaps for the first time, experienced what it feels like to live with greater clarity, energy, and inner alignment. But as you probably already sense, healing isn't just about the reset. It's about what happens next. This is where transformation becomes a way of living. Sustained transformation doesn't demand perfection — it requires integration. The truth is, the world you live in will keep pulling you back toward stress, convenience, numbness, and disconnection. It's wired that way. But you're no longer passive in that system. You're awake now. You've reconnected with your body's wisdom, and you've started building trust with it again. The question now becomes: how do you protect that connection? How do you live from it every day, without burning out, falling back into old patterns, or feeling like you have to fight to stay well?

This final part is about making your transformation stick — not through rigid discipline or chasing some flawless lifestyle, but through practices, mindsets, and shifts that are sustainable, soulful, and rooted in who you truly are. Because real health is not just about what you avoid or fix. It's about what you *embody*. It's about becoming the kind of person who lives with intention — who protects their energy, listens to their body, and makes decisions from a place of clarity, not chaos.

You'll learn how to protect the progress you've made — not with fear, but with discernment. You'll discover what it means to become the true authority of your health, how to advocate for yourself in a system that often dismisses real healing, and how to create simple daily rituals that nourish you without feeling like a burden. We'll explore what it looks like to fully live from a place of alignment — where your habits, thoughts, and environment support your vitality instead of undermining it.

Most importantly, this part of the journey is about moving beyond survival into creation. You're not here just to manage symptoms. You're here to *thrive*. To expand. To wake up each day feeling grounded in your body, confident in your choices, and connected to a vision for your life that actually excites you. That's what sustained transformation is: not a goal to chase, but a rhythm to live by.

You've already done the hardest part — you've started. Now let's make sure your reset becomes a lifestyle. One that lasts. One that uplifts. One that brings you home to yourself again and again.

Rewiring Your Beliefs Around Health

How Conditioning Keeps You Sick

Most of us don't realize just how much of our behavior is on autopilot. From what we eat to how we think about our symptoms, much of our daily life is shaped not by conscious choice — but by deep conditioning. And while some habits serve us, many others quietly sabotage our health. The danger isn't always in the overtly toxic substances or dramatic lifestyle choices. Often, it's the subtle, repetitive patterns — the ones that feel "normal" — that do the most damage over time.

Conditioning begins early. We're born into a world where food is marketed as pleasure and reward, rest is framed as laziness, and discomfort is something to be numbed. We're taught to seek quick fixes, to override the body's signals, and to defer to authority instead of tuning in to ourselves. By the time we reach adulthood, this programming is so ingrained that we don't question it. We don't even see it. It becomes the invisible operating system that runs our lives.

Take, for example, the way we handle fatigue. Instead of asking what the body might be trying to communicate, we're conditioned to reach for caffeine or sugar. Instead of resting, we push through. Over time, this disconnection from our natural rhythms contributes to burnout, hormone disruption, and immune dysfunction — all without us realizing we're doing anything "wrong." After all, everyone else is doing the same.

This social normalization is one of the most insidious aspects of conditioning. If everyone around you eats ultra-processed food, sleeps poorly, lives in a constant state of stress, and pops pills for symptoms, it's easy to assume this is just how life works. But the fact that something is common doesn't make it *natural*. Or healthy. It just means the conditioning has been successful.

Another layer of this programming comes from the medical system itself. Many of us were taught to believe that health is something only a professional can interpret. That our symptoms aren't valid unless they show up on a test. That being told "everything looks fine" — even when you feel far from it — means you must be imagining things. This creates a subtle but powerful fracture in your sense of self-trust. Over time, it teaches you to ignore your instincts, to second-guess your body, and to wait for permission to act.

Even wellness culture, despite its good intentions, can reinforce this conditioning. The endless stream of "biohacks," strict protocols, and trendy solutions often sends the same message: you're broken, and you need something *out there* to fix you. This keeps people stuck in a loop of chasing external solutions while still feeling fundamentally disconnected from their own body's wisdom.

But the truth is, real healing starts when we begin to decondition — when we become aware of the messages we've absorbed and start questioning them. Not with judgment, but with curiosity. Why do you feel guilty resting? Why do you assume discomfort must be numbed? Why do you trust a lab result more than the chronic fatigue you live with every day? These aren't just philosophical questions. They're the starting point of reclaiming your power.

As we peel back the layers of this conditioning, it becomes clear that staying sick isn't always about lack of knowledge — it's often about what we've been taught to ignore, dismiss, or accept. Now we'll explore exactly how to begin breaking these mental and behavioral patterns so you can step out of survival mode and into conscious health ownership.

So how do we begin to break free from this invisible grip that shapes our choices, often without us realizing?

The first step is awareness. Not dramatic action, not overhauling your entire life — just becoming aware. When you reach for the same snack every afternoon, pause and ask: am I hungry, or is this just a habit? When you feel the familiar twinge of anxiety and instinctively pick up your phone or open a browser tab, ask: what am I avoiding feeling? Noticing without judgment is the beginning of change. Conditioning thrives in the shadows — shine light on it, and it begins to lose power.

The second step is to slow down. Our culture rewards speed, productivity, and hustle. But healing doesn't happen in that environment. It requires space — to listen, to reflect, to reconnect. You don't need to go on a retreat or disappear into the mountains. Just start with a few quiet minutes in the morning. Observe your thoughts. Listen to your breath. Feel what your body is asking for. Over time, this kind of stillness allows buried messages to surface — and when they do, you'll start making decisions from a place of intuition, not programming.

It's also important to reclaim language. Pay attention to the words you use to describe your health. Do you say things like "I'm just getting old" or "It runs in my family"? These statements, often repeated without thought, reinforce helplessness. They reflect beliefs you've likely inherited, not truths you've chosen. Start shifting them. Try saying, "My body is speaking to me" instead of "Something's wrong with me." Or, "I'm learning how to support myself better," instead of "I guess I'm just broken." Language isn't just expression — it's programming. The words you choose shape how you think, and how you think shapes what you allow yourself to experience.

As you begin to unlearn what has been drilled into you for years, there may be resistance. That's normal. You might feel doubt. You might hear an inner voice whisper, "Who do you think you are to question this?" That's part of the old script fighting to stay relevant. Let it come. Acknowledge it. But don't let it drive.

Another critical part of deconditioning is to redefine what health actually means to you. The mainstream model defines it narrowly — mostly by numbers on a chart or how silent your symptoms are. But what if health wasn't just the absence of disease? What if it was the presence of vitality, mental clarity, deep rest, and the ability to experience life fully? What if it included emotional resilience, spiritual connection, and a sense of groundedness in your own body? When you expand your definition of health, you open up a whole new path for how to approach it — and you stop chasing someone else's idea of wellness.

The more you challenge the script, the more empowered you become. You stop living reactively. You stop waiting for a diagnosis to justify your fatigue or a prescription to validate your pain. You begin to trust your own signals and respond with integrity. That's the shift from passive patient to conscious participant. And it changes everything.

Finally, it's important to surround yourself with a new form of conditioning — one that supports your healing. Choose your inputs carefully. Curate your environment to include voices that reinforce your agency, your wisdom, and your potential for regeneration. That might mean spending less time around people who normalize burnout or ridicule your choices — and more time around those who are walking a similar path of reconnection.

It might mean choosing books, podcasts, and conversations that remind you: healing is possible, and it starts within.

This isn't about perfection. It's about waking up from the trance and deciding — again and again — to live in alignment with what your body truly needs. Conditioning can be unlearned. And once it is, you realize something powerful: you were never broken. You were just taught to ignore your own brilliance.

Healing begins the moment you remember who you were before the world taught you to forget. And from that place — of remembering — your reset truly begins.

Choosing Empowerment Over Fear

There comes a point on every healing journey when you face a decision —
one that quietly determines whether you'll continue circling the same
struggles or step into something radically different. That decision is whether
you will keep living from fear... or start choosing empowerment.

Most of us are conditioned to act from fear without even realizing it. We
fear symptoms. We fear diagnoses. We fear getting worse, being judged,
making the wrong choices, being too late, not knowing enough, or not being
"healthy" enough. This fear isn't always loud — sometimes it hides behind
logic, or responsibility, or even the desire to "do the right thing." But fear-
based living often shows up as over-researching, over-supplementing,
obsessing over food labels, or constantly second-guessing what our body is
telling us.

You might recognize the pattern: You feel off. Something's not right. You
immediately dive into search engines, forums, influencers, protocols. You
gather advice from every angle. And instead of feeling more informed, you
end up paralyzed. You've gathered so many opinions that you don't know
which way is up. Every decision feels like a potential mistake. Every step
forward feels heavy with doubt. That's fear in disguise — disguised as
"responsibility" or "trying to be informed."

But the truth is, healing doesn't happen in fear. Fear triggers survival mode
— biologically, emotionally, and energetically. When you operate from fear,
your body tightens. Your digestion slows. Your nervous system stays alert
and defensive. Your thoughts become scattered, your sleep becomes
shallow, and your connection to intuition goes offline. Even if you're doing
all the "right" things — eating clean, taking the best supplements,
exercising, meditating — if you're doing them from fear, your body still
perceives a threat. And that perception alone is enough to short-circuit
healing.

That's why empowerment matters.

Empowerment isn't about pretending everything is fine. It's not blind
optimism or spiritual bypassing. It's about choosing to stand in your own
authority, even when things feel uncertain. It's about acknowledging fear
without letting it control your actions. It's learning to say, "Yes, I don't have
all the answers — and I still trust my ability to respond."

Empowerment invites a different kind of energy into the healing process. It says: "My body is not my enemy. My symptoms are not punishments. I am not broken. I am learning. I am evolving." These aren't just affirmations — they're a shift in posture. They allow you to step out of panic and into curiosity. Out of victimhood and into agency.

This shift is subtle but powerful. It begins when you stop chasing health out of fear of disease and start pursuing vitality out of love for life. When you stop acting from a place of fixing what's wrong and start responding to what your body is asking for, moment by moment.

And yes — sometimes fear still shows up. That's normal. But instead of letting it drive, you learn to listen without reacting. You let it speak without obeying. Over time, it becomes background noise, no longer the main narrator of your journey.

This is where we pause — because the next part is learning how to *build that empowerment into your everyday decisions*. How do you shift from fear to trust, not just once, but repeatedly? How do you recognize when you're being pulled back into the old patterns? And how do you anchor yourself in your own inner compass, no matter what the world is telling you?

Let's explore.

Empowerment begins with presence. You can't choose differently if you don't notice the moment fear steps in. The first step is becoming aware — not just of the fear itself, but how it feels in your body. Does your chest tighten? Do your thoughts start to race? Do you feel the need to act immediately, fix something, or get certainty *now*? These sensations are cues. When you recognize them, you can pause. And in that pause, you reclaim your power.

From there, you begin to rewrite the script.

Instead of reacting, you respond. You take a breath and ask, "Is this decision coming from trust or from fear?" You ask yourself what *you* believe, not what the loudest voice on social media is saying. You learn to trust the messages of your body — not blindly, but with curiosity. Empowerment doesn't mean you never ask for help. It means you don't give away your authority when you do. You listen, you consider, but you filter everything through your own discernment.

This process becomes a daily practice. Choosing empowerment isn't a one-time event; it's a lifestyle. It's in the way you respond to new symptoms. The way you approach doctor visits. The way you talk to yourself on the hard days. And it's especially present in how you handle setbacks. Because healing isn't linear — there will be moments that challenge you. Symptoms may flare, plans may fall through, energy may dip. The old narrative will tempt you back: "Something's wrong. I'm failing. I need to control this." That's when the real work begins.

In those moments, empowerment looks like this: "I'm still safe. My body is adapting. This is not the end of the story." You stay grounded in the truth that healing is a relationship, not a checklist. And like any relationship, it deepens with attention, patience, and love.

You'll also notice how empowerment changes your interactions with others. When you're no longer seeking validation for every choice, you stop needing people to agree with you. You stop defending your path. You begin to speak more confidently, even when you're still figuring things out. You create boundaries that protect your peace. You become less reactive to fear-driven conversations — because you've already chosen a different operating system.

This doesn't mean you won't still feel vulnerable. True empowerment includes humility. It's okay to not have all the answers. It's okay to pivot, to try something new, to admit when something isn't working. That's not failure — it's wisdom. And it keeps you in a state of flexibility, which is essential for healing. Rigidity is a form of control. Flexibility is a sign of trust.

Eventually, something beautiful happens: your body starts to feel this shift. Not just mentally or emotionally, but physically. Your nervous system begins to relax. Your digestion improves. Sleep becomes deeper. Hormones begin to stabilize. Because when the body no longer has to brace against fear, it can finally begin to restore.

And in this state, you become magnetic. People may ask you what changed. They may see a softness in your face, a steadiness in your tone, a new glow in your eyes. It's not because you found the "perfect" protocol. It's because you stopped abandoning yourself.

That's what choosing empowerment really is — a return. A return to your own center. To your own body. To your own wisdom.

So if you ever find yourself slipping into fear again, don't judge it. Just pause. Come back to your breath. Remember that you have a choice in how you respond. That choice — quiet and powerful — is where your healing begins. And it's where it continues, one empowered moment at a time.

Breaking Free from the 'Fix-Me' Mentality

There's a quiet script running in the background of modern health culture, and it goes something like this: *You're broken. Something is wrong with you. You need someone to fix it.* Most people don't consciously adopt this narrative, but it's deeply embedded in the way we talk about health, illness, and healing. From the earliest signs of discomfort, we're conditioned to outsource — to look for pills, procedures, or professionals to solve the problem *for* us. This is the "fix-me" mentality, and it's one of the most disempowering frameworks we can carry.

At first glance, the desire to be "fixed" seems reasonable. If you're in pain, if you're exhausted, if your body feels like it's working against you, of course you want relief. Of course you want to feel better. But the deeper issue is this: the fix-me mentality places the power entirely outside of yourself. It reduces your body to a broken machine, your symptoms to glitches, and your role in healing to that of a passive observer.

This dynamic is reinforced everywhere — in the way doctors rush through appointments, in how medications are marketed, even in how we describe ourselves. "I have a bad gut," "My hormones are a mess," "I'm just genetically prone to fatigue." These statements may feel like truth, but they subtly reinforce the idea that something is inherently flawed in us — and that the solution lies elsewhere.

But what if the body isn't broken? What if symptoms aren't signs of malfunction, but intelligent signals? What if healing isn't something done *to* you, but something awakened *within* you?

These aren't just abstract ideas. They represent a fundamental shift in how we relate to our health. Breaking free from the fix-me mentality means moving from passivity to partnership. It's not about rejecting help — it's about reclaiming agency. It's understanding that your body is not a problem to be solved, but a system that responds to the inputs it's given — food, rest, emotions, stress, beliefs.

Many people get stuck because they're looking for the "one thing" that will fix them — the perfect supplement, the newest protocol, the right diagnosis. And while these tools can be useful, they often become distractions from the deeper truth: healing is a process that unfolds through connection, not correction. It's not about doing more, but about listening more deeply.

You may find yourself wondering, "If I'm not broken, then why do I feel so unwell?" That's a valid question. But feeling unwell is not proof of brokenness. It's proof that something needs your attention. It may be that your body is overwhelmed, undernourished, inflamed, or carrying years of unprocessed stress. These are real challenges — but they're not evidence that you're defective. They're signs that your body is still trying, still communicating, still working for you.

This realization can be confronting. It means letting go of the fantasy that someone else can save you. It means no longer waiting for permission or perfection to begin. But it also means something far more liberating: you get to stop fighting your body. You get to start working with it.

This is where the shift truly begins — in that moment when you stop asking "What's wrong with me?" and begin asking, "What is my body trying to tell me?"

The truth is, your body is not your enemy. It's your most loyal ally. Even when it feels like it's betraying you — through fatigue, bloating, pain, or fog — it's actually speaking in the only language it knows. The challenge is that most of us were never taught how to listen. We were taught to silence the symptoms, to suppress the discomfort, and to override the messages with quick fixes.

But real healing begins when we stop trying to mute the body and start decoding it.

Think about how often we wait to make changes until something becomes unbearable. We tolerate the mild symptoms, dismiss the fatigue, normalize the headaches. And when the body finally screams — with a diagnosis, a breakdown, or a chronic condition — we say, "Now I need to be fixed." But the body was never malfunctioning. It was just whispering for years before it finally had to shout.

Breaking free from the fix-me mindset requires a shift in how we define progress. It's no longer about chasing an end result — the perfect body, the absence of symptoms, the glowing health image we've been sold. Instead, it's about building a relationship with your body that's rooted in trust. One where you show up consistently, not out of fear, but out of respect.

This kind of relationship isn't built overnight. It starts with small acts of listening. Asking yourself, "How do I feel after eating this?" or "What happens when I sleep less than seven hours?" It's in noticing how your body responds to stress, or how certain environments drain you while others restore you. It's in choosing food, movement, and rest not because someone said you *should*, but because your body clearly responds well to them.

This also means rejecting the idea that health must be earned through suffering. You don't need to punish your body into wellness. You don't need to "detox" it through deprivation or force it into rigid routines. These approaches are often rooted in the same mindset: that something is wrong with you, and it must be controlled or corrected. True healing, in contrast, is rooted in nourishment, not restriction.

You are not a problem to be solved. You are a whole, intelligent being — and your body reflects that intelligence. When something is off, it's not a sign of failure, but an invitation to inquire. It's a call to become curious, compassionate, and collaborative with your own physiology.

Some people resist this idea because it feels too simple. "What do you mean I just need to listen to my body?" they ask. But simplicity doesn't mean easy. Listening — truly listening — is one of the hardest things we do, especially in a world that constantly teaches us to override intuition and obey authority.

And yet, this is the foundation of sustained transformation. When you shift from needing to be fixed to trusting your body's guidance, something profound happens. You stop chasing. You start aligning. You begin to recognize patterns and break cycles. You become less reactive and more intentional. You stop waiting for someone else to rescue you — and start becoming the steward of your own health.

This doesn't mean you'll never seek help or guidance again. There's a difference between support and dependency. The goal isn't isolation; it's sovereignty. It's knowing that even when you work with others — doctors, coaches, nutritionists — you're not handing over your power. You're collaborating with them, not surrendering to them.

Ultimately, the path forward isn't about fixing. It's about remembering. Remembering that your body is wise. That it wants to heal. That healing is not about perfection — it's about presence.

You're not here to be fixed. You're here to reconnect. And that shift alone is enough to change everything.

Food as Intelligence, Not Just Fuel

Beyond Calories: Food as Communication

For most of us, food has been reduced to numbers — calories in, calories out. Carbs are demonized, fats are feared, protein is glorified, and we track every bite with apps, charts, and portion sizes. Somewhere along the way, the living language of food was lost. We stopped seeing meals as nourishment and started treating them like math problems. But food is far more than a tally of macros and calories — it's a form of communication between you and your body, between your body and your environment, and between your cells and their future.

Every bite of food carries information. Not just nutrients, but instructions. When you eat, you're not simply fueling your body — you're sending it messages. Messages that can either trigger inflammation or reduce it. Messages that can support hormonal balance or disrupt it. Messages that can nurture the gut or damage it.

Let's take a simple example: when you eat a fresh salad full of leafy greens, colorful vegetables, healthy fats, and maybe some fermented elements, you're delivering signals that support your microbiome, calm your nervous system, and nourish your mitochondria. Compare that to a heavily processed fast-food meal. Your body still receives the food — but the message is very different. That message might say: "We're in survival mode," "Prepare for stress," or "Inflammation incoming."

Your body doesn't think in terms of calories. It responds to biochemical cues. It notices the presence of pesticides, artificial additives, preservatives, and excess sugar. It pays attention to fiber, polyphenols, and naturally occurring enzymes. These signals influence everything — your metabolism, mood, immune function, and even gene expression. This is why two meals with the same caloric content can have completely opposite effects on your body's systems.

And it goes deeper than nutrients. The *quality* of the food matters — not just what you eat, but where it came from, how it was grown, how it was cooked, and how it was consumed. A tomato ripened under the sun in rich, living soil speaks a different biochemical language than one grown in nutrient-depleted ground, picked unripe, and gassed to look red on the shelf. Your body knows the difference, even if you don't consciously register it.

But we've been trained to ignore that language. We've been told to count, to restrict, to substitute, to hack — as though our bodies were machines and food was fuel. That industrial, mechanical model of health has led us far from the intuitive understanding that food is *information*. And not all information is benign.

This disconnect is one reason why so many people feel like they're doing "everything right" and still not seeing results. They're eating within their calorie limits. They're avoiding certain macros. But they're still inflamed, exhausted, and imbalanced — because the body doesn't just want fuel. It wants messages it can trust.

Now, before we dive deeper, this isn't a call to obsess over every bite or to moralize food choices. This isn't about "good" or "bad" food — it's about clear or confusing messages. It's about understanding that your body is always listening, and food is one of the most direct ways we speak to it.

That brings us to a powerful shift: what happens when we stop micromanaging numbers and start tuning into the dialogue?

If food is a language, then every meal is a conversation. And like any conversation, the tone matters. When we eat in a rush, distracted, stressed, or emotionally checked out, we change not just how we digest the food — but how the message is received by our body. Digestion doesn't begin in the stomach; it starts in the mind. The signals we send through breath, posture, and attention all influence how our body handles what comes next. This is why ancient cultures often incorporated prayer, gratitude, or ritual before meals. It wasn't superstition. It was biology. Taking a moment to breathe, to acknowledge the nourishment, to slow down — that's a signal to the body that it's safe. Safe to rest. Safe to digest. Safe to repair. In contrast, eating while scrolling through your phone or driving in traffic sends a very different message: one of stress and alertness. And when you're in a state of stress, digestion is deprioritized, absorption suffers, and inflammation rises.

But there's another piece to this — our emotional relationship with food. For many people, food is no longer about nourishment at all. It's about control, guilt, punishment, reward, and comfort. We use it to soothe wounds we haven't yet faced. We restrict it when we feel the need to reclaim control. We binge when we're overwhelmed. In doing so, we send our bodies mixed messages — confusion, chaos, and inconsistency.

This isn't just about the body — it's about the self. If we constantly approach food from a place of fear — fear of gaining weight, of eating "wrong," of not doing enough — then we create a feedback loop of anxiety. And the body doesn't thrive in anxiety. Healing doesn't happen when we're in fight-or-flight. It happens when we feel grounded, safe, and nourished. When food becomes a source of fear or shame, it loses its healing power, no matter how "clean" the ingredients are.

So the work of restoring health is not just about what's on the plate — it's about the intention behind it. It's asking: *What am I telling my body right now?* Am I telling it to brace for war, or to lean into healing? Am I signaling trust or punishment? Connection or disconnection?

When you begin to shift the way you see food — from numbers to language, from fear to relationship — something remarkable happens. You start to make different choices, not because you have to, but because they feel aligned. You begin to crave foods that nourish you instead of depleting you. You notice how different your body feels when you eat with intention, when you slow down, when you listen.

You also start to see through the noise. You're no longer pulled into every new trend or restrictive plan that promises quick fixes. Instead, you recognize that the real power lies in *how* you eat, not just *what* you eat. This is how the body heals — not through control, but through clarity. Not through rigid rules, but through honest communication.

And perhaps most importantly, you stop outsourcing your power. You stop giving your agency away to apps, charts, influencers, or even experts. You begin to trust your own feedback. You begin to recognize that your body isn't broken — it's intelligent. It's been waiting for you to listen. And food is one of the clearest ways it speaks.

In the end, food is not a battleground. It's not punishment or salvation. It's dialogue. It's connection. It's information. And when you start treating it as such — with respect, with curiosity, and with care — you change not just your health, but your entire relationship with yourself. That's when healing begins. Not just on a cellular level, but on a soul-deep one.

How to Eat to Stay Clear, Strong, and Resilient

We've been taught to eat for survival. For weight control. For calories in, calories out. But what if we shifted the question from "how do I eat to stay thin?" to "how do I eat to stay powerful, clear-minded, and resilient in a world that often drains me?"

That shift changes everything.

Because food is more than fuel — it's the foundation of your internal environment. It influences how you feel, how you think, how you handle stress, how well you sleep, and how fast you bounce back. If you're foggy, anxious, bloated, or exhausted, there's a high chance your food choices are contributing — not just because of what you eat, but how and why you eat it.

The truth is, the body doesn't just need nutrients — it needs signals. And food sends signals to your biology every time you eat. It can either amplify inflammation or calm it. It can either activate your stress pathways or support your rest-and-digest systems. It can either contribute to hormonal chaos or help restore hormonal balance. That's the power you hold, every single day.

Let's start with clarity. If your mind feels heavy, cloudy, or reactive, it's often a sign that something in your internal chemistry is off. That doesn't mean you need a stimulant — it means you need stability. Sugar spikes, ultra-processed foods, and chemical additives may give you temporary energy, but they come with a cost: mental crashes, irritability, and eventually, chronic fatigue. Eating to stay clear means reducing the noise — literally. Simplifying your meals, prioritizing whole foods, and minimizing ingredients you can't pronounce is a simple but powerful strategy. Your brain thrives on clean, steady input — not chaos.

Strength, on the other hand, is not just about muscle. It's about cellular strength — the ability of your body to function under pressure and not fall apart. That means supporting your mitochondria (your body's energy generators), your nervous system, and your digestion. To do that, your meals need to be rich in micronutrients, not just macros. Think of foods that come from the earth — unaltered, unrefined, alive. These are the foods your body recognizes. And when your body recognizes what's coming in, it knows how to use it. This translates into better recovery, less inflammation, and greater physical vitality.

Then there's resilience — your ability to return to balance after being challenged. In today's world, we're bombarded daily by stressors, pollutants, inflammatory triggers, and emotional tension. Resilience isn't about avoiding hardship. It's about how fast you recover. And that recovery depends heavily on your internal environment — which means your food habits matter more than most people realize. If you're constantly eating on autopilot, reaching for what's fast or addictive, your body stays stuck in survival mode. But when you begin eating in a way that prioritizes nourishment, stability, and calm, your body starts to shift back toward equilibrium — and from that place, real resilience becomes possible.

None of this is about perfection. This isn't a restrictive diet or another wellness trend. It's a mindset — a long-term strategy that honors your biology instead of overriding it. It's learning how to choose foods that *speak the same language* as your body. Because when that language aligns, everything changes — from your energy to your immunity, your clarity to your sense of self.

So how do you bring this into your everyday life — in a world where food is everywhere, time is short, and convenience often wins?

The first shift is presence. That means slowing down enough to actually notice what you're choosing and why. Most people eat reactively — out of habit, boredom, stress, or emotional patterning. But when you eat with awareness, you reclaim choice. You begin to ask yourself: Will this meal help me feel grounded or scattered? Energized or drained? Nourished or numbed out?

Once you start asking that question, everything softens. The pressure to be "perfect" falls away, and what's left is something much more sustainable: a daily commitment to choosing what serves your clarity and strength. Not every meal will be ideal. That's okay. What matters is the pattern you create over time.

In practice, this means leaning into simplicity. Meals made from whole, real ingredients — ones your grandmother would recognize — tend to support your body better than anything wrapped in layers of plastic and loaded with synthetic additives. But it's not just about cutting things out. It's about remembering what to include. Fresh vegetables, good fats, clean protein, and grounding complex carbohydrates — these aren't trendy. They're foundational. When they become the baseline of your eating, your body starts to come back to life.

Equally important is the rhythm of eating. Many people either graze all day or skip meals entirely, leaving their body confused and stressed. Your body likes rhythm. It responds well to regular nourishment, not only in content but in timing. Eating at roughly consistent intervals supports hormonal balance, blood sugar stability, and a more even emotional tone. It helps your nervous system trust that it's not constantly in survival mode.

But even more subtle — and more powerful — is how you feel when you eat. If you're always rushing, scrolling, or multitasking, your body doesn't register the meal properly. Digestion starts before your first bite. It begins with your attention. Taking a breath before a meal, sitting down without distractions, and chewing slowly can radically change how food is processed. It allows your parasympathetic nervous system — the "rest and digest" mode — to activate, which not only improves nutrient absorption but also reduces inflammation and digestive distress.

Then there's hydration. Often overlooked, it plays a quiet but essential role in clarity and resilience. The brain is around 75% water. Even mild dehydration can impair concentration, energy, and mood. But hydration isn't just about drinking water — it's about balance. Including electrolytes, minerals, and hydrating foods like fruits and vegetables helps your cells actually use the water you drink. A dry, processed diet — even if it's calorie-dense — can leave the body chronically dehydrated at the cellular level. That kind of dehydration doesn't just impact performance; it wears you down emotionally, too.

As you move toward this more intentional way of eating, you may notice resistance — both internally and externally. You may hear voices telling you it's too much work, or that you'll never be consistent. You might feel social pressure to keep eating the way others around you do. That's normal. And it's part of the process. But the truth is, when you experience what it feels like to eat in a way that supports your nervous system, your gut, and your energy — it becomes almost impossible to go back.

This isn't about diet culture. It's not about food rules or guilt. It's about building a relationship with your body that's rooted in care, respect, and long-term vitality. The more aligned your eating becomes with your biology, the more you begin to *trust* your body again — and that trust is the foundation of lasting transformation.

You are not meant to feel foggy, weak, or burned out. Your body was designed for resilience. The food you eat each day can either anchor that resilience or erode it — and every meal is a new opportunity to choose your strength.

The Foods That Heal vs. The Foods That Steal

Every bite you take is either contributing to your healing or pulling you further from it. This may sound dramatic, but when you look closely at how the body responds to food — hormonally, neurologically, and at the cellular level — it becomes clear: food is not neutral. It communicates. It directs. It either supports your natural vitality or gradually depletes it.

Yet for most people, this connection between food and well-being has been dulled. We've grown up in a culture where eating is often divorced from nourishment. Where cravings are manufactured, not intuitive. Where "normal" eating patterns are based more on convenience, marketing, and habit than actual physiological need. And where foods that harm are not only legal, but aggressively promoted.

Let's start with the foods that steal — not just your energy, but your clarity, your balance, your ability to heal. These are the ultra-processed staples of the modern diet: refined sugars, industrial seed oils, synthetic additives, hormone-disrupting preservatives, and hyper-palatable junk that floods the system with chemical signals the body was never designed to process. These substances don't simply pass through; they affect mood, disrupt the gut-brain axis, spike blood sugar, suppress immune function, and over time, lay the foundation for chronic inflammation.

And the problem isn't just what's in these foods. It's also what they displace. When processed foods dominate the diet, healing foods are pushed aside. Whole vegetables, clean fats, fermented foods, mineral-rich broths, antioxidant-packed herbs — these rarely coexist with drive-thru dinners or grab-and-go energy bars. You can't build a resilient body on a foundation of synthetic calories and hope that supplements will patch the gaps. It doesn't work that way.

But when you start reintroducing real, healing foods — slowly, steadily — you begin to feel the shift. Your body isn't confused by these foods. It recognizes them. It knows what to do with them. And often, it responds faster than expected.

Healing foods aren't trendy or exotic. They're often simple, ancestral, and consistent with what humans have always eaten in times of health. Think deeply colored vegetables, nutrient-dense roots, pasture-raised proteins, omega-3-rich seafood, herbs that have been used for centuries in traditional medicine. These foods speak the language of your cells. They soothe the gut

114

lining, stabilize blood sugar, support detox pathways, and help reset the nervous system from chronic alert.

For example, the fiber in vegetables and fruits isn't just "good for digestion." It feeds beneficial gut bacteria that in turn regulate everything from mood to immune response. The fats in wild-caught salmon or cold-pressed olive oil aren't just fuel — they form the very structure of your brain cells and stabilize inflammation. The sulfur compounds in garlic, the polyphenols in berries, the curcumin in turmeric — these aren't nutrients your body treats passively. They are active agents of repair.

There's no need to obsess or over-restrict. But clarity matters. If you know a certain food is consistently making you feel worse, it's worth asking why. If a "treat" leaves you bloated, foggy, anxious, or wired, is it really a treat? If your morning coffee and pastry are followed by a blood sugar crash and low-grade anxiety, that's information — not punishment. And it's in that awareness that the shift begins.

This isn't about eliminating every indulgence or living in fear of ingredients. It's about waking up to what your body has likely been trying to tell you for years.

Learning to eat in a way that supports healing isn't about adhering to someone else's rigid food philosophy. It's about restoring a lost dialogue between your body and the food it actually thrives on. That process doesn't start with discipline — it starts with listening. Noticing how you feel after certain meals, how your energy responds, how your sleep shifts, how your skin looks, how your gut behaves. These small signals are your body's language. And they're often clearer than lab results.

The healing path is less about perfection and more about momentum. You don't need to eat clean 100% of the time to feel better. But what you do need is honesty. If your day-to-day habits revolve around foods that drain you, numb you, or trigger inflammatory responses, it's time to recalibrate. That doesn't mean eliminating everything at once. It means making conscious choices to reduce the volume of what steals from you and increase the volume of what heals you.

Start simple. Replace the packaged snacks that leave you sluggish with something vibrant and alive. Swap your usual sugar-loaded breakfast with something that stabilizes your blood sugar and sets the tone for the day.

Bring in one new healing food each week — not because you have to, but because you're curious about how your body might respond.

Remember that food is not just fuel. It's instruction. When you eat food that supports your gut microbiome, that nourishes your mitochondria, that reduces systemic inflammation, you're not just eating — you're sending messages to every cell in your body. Messages that say: you're safe, you're supported, you can heal now.

The modern diet, by contrast, often sends the opposite message. Constant blood sugar spikes keep your nervous system on high alert. Artificial additives and pesticide residues confuse your detox pathways. Low-nutrient meals leave your body hunting for missing pieces. And then we wonder why anxiety, fatigue, chronic pain, and hormonal chaos are so widespread. These aren't random glitches. They're biological consequences.

We can't talk about healing foods without acknowledging how heavily the deck is stacked against them in today's food landscape. Ultra-processed products are cheaper, more convenient, and aggressively marketed — especially to the most vulnerable. They are designed not to nourish but to hijack your taste buds and override your natural satiety cues. Many of them are legally food, but biologically toxic.

This is why food isn't just a personal choice — it's a form of quiet rebellion. When you choose to nourish instead of numb, to energize instead of suppress, to heal instead of cope, you're stepping outside of a system that profits from your disconnection. You're reclaiming authority over your own biology.

And that's the deeper truth behind the phrase "food is medicine." It's not a slogan. It's a biological reality. The compounds in whole foods interact with your body in intelligent, nuanced ways. They regulate inflammation, repair tissue, balance hormones, and modulate immunity. You don't need exotic superfoods or expensive supplements to tap into this. You need consistency, quality, and a willingness to let go of the false comfort that toxic food provides.

The shift begins when food becomes a conversation again. Not a battle, not a rulebook, but a living relationship. When you learn to feed your body in a way that affirms life, the changes are often undeniable. Clarity returns. Energy steadies. Bloating fades. Sleep deepens. And perhaps most importantly, you stop feeling like your body is your enemy. You begin to feel — often for the first time in years — that your body is working with you, not against you.

Healing doesn't have to be complicated. But it does have to be intentional. The foods you choose are among the most consistent decisions you make every single day. With each meal, you're either reinforcing health or eroding it. Not in a fearful, perfectionist way — but in a real, biochemical way that matters more than you've probably been told.

And now, you know better. So your choices can be different. More aligned. More powerful. More alive. Because healing isn't a future destination. It's something you begin to build — one conscious meal at a time.

Emotional & Energetic Health

Stress, Stored Trauma, and Their Physical Toll

We've been taught to separate the mind from the body — to treat emotional struggles as one thing and physical symptoms as another. But that division is an illusion. Your body doesn't compartmentalize in the way Western medicine often does. It records everything. Every moment of stress, every unresolved trauma, every emotional upheaval — it's all imprinted in the nervous system, the gut, the tissues, and even the immune response.

Stress is not just a feeling; it's a full-body event. When you experience it, even in small doses, your body shifts into a state of vigilance. Your heart rate increases. Cortisol floods your bloodstream. Digestion slows. Your immune system is temporarily put on hold. This is a survival mechanism — meant to protect you in short bursts. But when stress becomes chronic, your body gets stuck in survival mode, and over time, this wears you down.

The trouble is that most people don't realize how stressed they are until the symptoms become undeniable. It doesn't always look like panic or high blood pressure. It often looks like constant fatigue, trouble sleeping, gut discomfort, or random aches and pains that don't seem to have a cause. It shows up in hormone imbalances, low-grade inflammation, or autoimmune flare-ups. This isn't weakness. It's biology.

And it's not just about what's happening now. Past trauma — especially the kind that wasn't fully processed — can stay lodged in the body, silently affecting how your nervous system operates today. This is why some people seem to live with a constant undercurrent of tension or unease, even when life seems stable on the surface. Their body has learned to expect danger, even in the absence of it. This is what's often referred to as "stored trauma" — and its effects are real.

Stored trauma doesn't always come from major events. It can arise from subtle but chronic experiences: childhood emotional neglect, unstable environments, repeated betrayals, or long-term exposure to stress that felt impossible to escape. Your body doesn't measure trauma by how dramatic the event was — it responds based on how overwhelmed you were and how much support you had to process what was happening. In the absence of that support, the experience stays unintegrated, and your nervous system holds onto it.

What this looks like in daily life can be complex. You might find yourself reacting strongly to minor stressors, struggling with motivation, or feeling disconnected from your body. You might experience digestive issues that don't resolve with diet alone. Or you might carry tension in your shoulders, jaw, or gut without realizing it — because that tension has become your baseline.

The link between unprocessed emotional experiences and physical health has been studied extensively, though it's still not widely acknowledged in mainstream healthcare. Research in the field of psychoneuroimmunology, for instance, shows that chronic stress and emotional trauma can alter immune function, increase inflammation, and even change gene expression. This is not about blame — it's about understanding the full picture of what health really requires.

If you've spent years chasing symptom relief without real resolution, it may be time to ask a deeper question: what has your body been holding onto that it never had the chance to release?

The body remembers what the mind tries to forget. And if the memory hasn't been metabolized — meaning it hasn't been processed, understood, or given space — it doesn't just fade away. It lingers in the background, influencing how your body functions and how your brain responds to the world around you. Over time, this can create a kind of internal static, a chronic state of dysregulation that no supplement or green smoothie can fully resolve on its own.

This is where true healing asks for a shift in approach. Instead of simply trying to manage or suppress symptoms, we begin to ask what the body is trying to communicate. Fatigue might not be a flaw in your energy system — it might be a signal that you've been carrying too much for too long. Chronic tension might not be a posture issue — it could be your body's attempt to stay braced for danger that's no longer present. Digestive dysfunction might not be just about food — it could be your gut responding to a lifetime of nervous system overload.

This is not a call to pathologize your emotions, nor to believe that everything physical is "just trauma." That would be another kind of oversimplification. But it is a call to look more closely — to consider the

119

whole of your story, not just the list of symptoms. Because the more you understand what's underneath your physical distress, the more power you have to address it at the root.

There is a reason why practices like breathwork, somatic therapy, meditation, and even mindful movement are increasingly recognized not as fringe, but foundational. They help regulate a dysregulated nervous system. They create space for stored trauma to surface safely, be witnessed, and be released. They shift your body from survival to restoration — from fight-or-flight to repair-and-rebuild.

But these shifts don't come instantly. Releasing stored trauma isn't like draining a tank. It's more like slowly melting ice. The body lets go only when it feels safe enough to do so. That's why healing can feel slow or uneven — and why it often requires more than logic. You can't think your way out of chronic stress. You have to feel your way through it. Gently, patiently, and with deep respect for what your body has endured.

As you begin to peel back these layers, you might notice changes that seem unrelated at first — like sleeping better, feeling more grounded, having less pain, or even experiencing more emotional resilience. That's not a coincidence. That's your body responding to a new environment: one in which it no longer has to be on high alert all the time.

It's important to emphasize that healing isn't about reliving the past or diving headfirst into emotional pain. It's about creating conditions where your nervous system learns a new baseline — one where calm is familiar, not foreign. Where connection, rather than protection, becomes your default. Where the body is no longer a battlefield but a home you can trust again.

This work is both subtle and powerful. And while it may not offer the immediate gratification that some health trends promise, it offers something far more valuable: long-term integrity. When you address the nervous system — when you tend to what's stored and suppressed — you make space for the body to do what it was always designed to do: repair, adapt, and return to balance.

Stress and trauma may have shaped your story, but they don't have to define it. You are not broken. You are a system doing its best to stay alive in a world that hasn't always made that easy. And once your body starts to feel safe, truly safe, healing stops being something you chase — and starts becoming something you embody.

Nervous System Reset & Emotional Hygiene

It's hard to heal in a body that's constantly on high alert. Even when we're not in immediate danger, many of us live as if we are. We rush through our days, flinch at every notification, and lie awake with our minds racing. We've normalized this state of overstimulation — and yet it's exactly this chronic dysregulation of the nervous system that quietly undermines our health.

Most people don't realize how central the nervous system is to their overall well-being. It's not just about how you respond to stress or how easily you relax — it's the master regulator of everything from digestion to hormones, immune response to mental clarity. When the nervous system is stuck in survival mode — whether from past trauma, environmental stressors, or daily overwhelm — the rest of the body follows its lead. Healing becomes difficult. Inflammation stays elevated. Hormones misfire. Sleep becomes fragmented. And no matter how clean your diet or how much you exercise, something still feels off.

That's because the body won't prioritize healing when it thinks it needs to defend itself. Even low-grade stress — the kind you carry quietly, without noticing — can keep the sympathetic nervous system (the fight-or-flight branch) dominant. This isn't a design flaw. It's biology. Your nervous system is built to protect you. But in today's world, that protection often backfires. We end up reacting to modern life as if it were a battlefield.

Resetting the nervous system isn't about doing more — it's about doing less, but with intention. It begins with interrupting the cycle of constant stimulation. This doesn't mean moving to a cabin in the woods or quitting your job. It means becoming aware of what pushes you into overdrive and what brings you back to calm. It's about learning to notice the cues your body gives you — the tight jaw, the shallow breath, the twitch in your stomach — and choosing not to override them.

One of the most profound yet overlooked parts of this reset is what could be called "emotional hygiene." Just like physical hygiene prevents infections and supports health, emotional hygiene helps prevent toxic emotional buildup — the kind that clogs your system and leaves you heavy, reactive, and exhausted. Most of us were never taught how to care for our emotions. We were taught to suppress them, analyze them, or distract ourselves from them. But emotions are messengers. If you don't process them, they don't disappear — they get stored.

And when they get stored without resolution, they begin to distort how we perceive life. We become quick to assume threat, slow to trust, and often disconnected from our true needs. Emotional hygiene is the practice of honoring these feelings, giving them space, and helping them move through the body instead of getting stuck. It's not dramatic or complex. Sometimes it looks like pausing to breathe when sadness wells up instead of swallowing it down. Sometimes it's letting yourself feel anger fully without turning it on someone else. Sometimes it's writing out the truth of what you feel without editing for politeness or logic.

This kind of practice builds internal spaciousness. And with space comes clarity, choice, and healing.

Resetting the nervous system doesn't demand perfection — it invites presence. The small, consistent ways you relate to your body and emotions throughout the day are what matter most. For many, the shift begins with breath. Not forced or structured breathing, but simply remembering to breathe all the way down into the belly. When your breath deepens, your nervous system gets the message: it's safe. You're not under threat. Your body can soften.

Equally important is the practice of pausing. In our culture, momentum is often mistaken for progress. We speed from one task to the next, thinking we're getting ahead, when in fact, we're just staying distracted. But it's in the pauses — those small moments between doing — where regulation is restored. It might be a few quiet minutes in your car before entering the house. Or standing at the sink and truly feeling the water on your hands. These are not "breaks from life." They are life, lived in the body.

Another key piece of nervous system healing is the way we move. While exercise is valuable, not all movement is created equal when it comes to regulation. Movement that's aggressive or disconnected from breath can actually reinforce a fight-or-flight pattern. What helps instead is movement that invites awareness back into the body — gentle stretching, walking without a destination, swaying to music, or even lying on the floor and feeling gravity hold you. When movement becomes a conversation with the body rather than a performance or punishment, the body feels met. And when it feels met, it relaxes its defenses.

On an emotional level, the reset comes when we stop judging what we feel. Emotions are not flaws in our design — they're how we metabolize experience. When sadness arises, it's a call for presence. When anger comes forward, it may be highlighting a boundary that was crossed. When fear surfaces, it could be asking for safety or clarity. The practice is not to force these feelings out but to be curious. To listen. To ask what they need.

One of the simplest and most effective ways to practice emotional hygiene is to let your feelings have form. That could mean writing them out — uncensored, without needing them to make sense. It could mean speaking them aloud when you're alone, giving them sound instead of silence. For some, it might mean naming the emotion in real-time: "This is grief. It's here. I'm not going to run from it." These small acts of acknowledgment prevent emotional stagnation, which is where so much of our tension, illness, and confusion arise.

It's also worth acknowledging that nervous system dysregulation and emotional suppression are often not just habits — they're adaptations. If you grew up in a home where feelings were unsafe, or if you've experienced trauma, your nervous system may have learned that being numb or constantly on guard was necessary. There's no shame in this. In fact, recognizing how intelligent those adaptations were is a form of healing in itself. But now, as an adult, you can offer your body something it may have never received: safety, softness, permission to feel without judgment.

There's no finish line in this work. No perfect nervous system. No badge for emotional mastery. There's only the ongoing relationship — between you and your body, your breath, your inner world. And with each choice to slow down, to soften, to feel, you're rewiring something profound. You're moving from survival into aliveness.

In the end, this isn't about controlling your nervous system or fixing your emotions. It's about building a container strong enough to hold your full human experience. And from that place, real healing becomes not only possible — it becomes inevitable.

How to Protect Your Energy Daily

You've probably felt it before — walking into a room and sensing tension before anyone says a word, or leaving a conversation with someone who barely talked but somehow feeling completely drained. This isn't just intuition or imagination. Your energy — the sum total of your physical vitality, emotional balance, mental clarity, and even your sense of spiritual alignment — is a real and measurable part of your health. And in today's world, it's constantly under pressure.

Most people don't think about energy as something to protect. We protect our homes with locks and our data with passwords, but we often leave our internal state wide open. We absorb stress from the news before we've even gotten out of bed. We get caught in cycles of comparison on social media. We overextend ourselves in relationships where giving is one-sided. And then we wonder why we feel exhausted, irritable, unfocused, or on edge.

Protecting your energy isn't about building walls or becoming hypervigilant. It's about becoming selective. Conscious. You're not obligated to carry the emotional burdens of others. You're not required to expose yourself to noise, conflict, or negativity in the name of staying "informed" or "polite." Your energetic boundaries deserve the same care and clarity as your physical ones.

This begins with awareness. The first and most important practice in energy protection is noticing what drains you — not in theory, but in real time. It might be a type of conversation, a place, a pattern of thinking, or even a time of day when you feel more vulnerable to overstimulation or emotional reactivity. Your body knows the answer before your mind does. Pay attention to that flutter in the chest, the tightness in the gut, the heaviness behind the eyes. These are not just sensations — they are signals.

Equally, notice what restores you. Not just the big things like vacations or spa days, but the small, quiet shifts that bring you back to yourself. A moment of stillness in the morning before your phone is on. A glass of water with lemon. Turning down the lights in the evening. Speaking kindly to yourself. These aren't indulgences — they're recalibrations. And they matter more than most people realize.

One powerful way to protect your energy is to begin each day with intention — not from a productivity standpoint, but from a sovereignty standpoint. Who do I want to be today? What energy do I want to embody? What do I want to carry, and what am I no longer available for? These questions anchor you. They give your nervous system a roadmap. Instead of reacting to everything that comes your way, you begin responding from a centered place. You stop letting the outside world decide how you feel inside.

This kind of presence can feel radical, especially in a culture that rewards overstimulation and speed. But it's not about withdrawing from life — it's about choosing how you engage with it. You can still be in the world, connected, responsive, and generous — while also remaining rooted in your own state. You can hold space for others without being consumed by their chaos. You can listen without absorbing. Support without self-sacrifice.

As you begin to cultivate this internal awareness and energetic clarity, you might notice that certain habits or relationships no longer feel sustainable. This is not a failure — it's a realignment. And it's often in these moments that we find the courage to set boundaries that are long overdue.

When you begin protecting your energy, life doesn't necessarily get quieter — but your internal response does. You stop being pulled into every emotional current around you. The noise doesn't stop, but your reaction to it softens. Instead of carrying everything, you start choosing what's truly yours. And that's where a profound sense of freedom begins.

One of the most powerful shifts in this process is recognizing that not every problem requires your involvement. Not every message demands a response. Not every invitation needs a yes. Your availability is not infinite. Your time, your attention, your nervous system — these are precious, finite resources. When you give them away too freely, your body eventually keeps the score. Fatigue, anxiety, mental fog — they are often symptoms of too much outward focus and too little inner preservation.

This is especially true in relationships. Energy protection doesn't mean becoming cold or distant. It means becoming honest. Are you constantly the one holding space for others, even when you're depleted? Do certain people leave you feeling energetically hijacked, as if you've just run a marathon after a simple conversation? These patterns are not small — they chip away at your vitality over time.

Sometimes, we avoid setting boundaries because we fear the reaction. But the truth is, the people who benefit most from your lack of boundaries are the ones most likely to resist them. That doesn't make your boundary wrong — it makes it necessary. And when you begin to stand in your own energetic clarity, you'll notice something subtle but life-changing: the right people respect it. The people who value your presence will also value your preservation.

Another crucial layer in daily energy protection is learning to close your own energy loops. Throughout the day, your system is exposed to hundreds of micro-interactions — moments of stimulation, challenge, or tension that don't always get resolved. These may seem insignificant, but your body holds onto them. A heated email, an unresolved conflict, even a tense encounter with a stranger can linger in your system long after the moment has passed.

To close these loops, you don't need elaborate rituals. You need honesty and attention. A few minutes of silence. A few deep breaths. Acknowledging what you're feeling instead of pushing it aside. Sometimes it's as simple as stepping outside and letting your nervous system reset in nature, or writing a sentence or two in a journal just to move the energy through. The key is to give yourself a space where your own experience can be seen and met — by you.

Over time, these practices compound. They become a quiet resilience — a strength that doesn't shout, but stands unshaken. You begin to move through the world with more discernment. You notice when a conversation is starting to drain you, and you choose to pause. You feel when a headline is designed to provoke, and you decide not to click. You sense when a part of your routine no longer aligns with your well-being, and you give yourself permission to let it go.

Protecting your energy daily isn't about control — it's about sovereignty. It's not about being perfect or rigid. It's about being present and anchored in yourself, so that you don't get swept up in energies that were never yours to carry.

As this awareness deepens, you may find that your entire relationship with "health" begins to shift. You start realizing that health isn't only about what you eat, how you move, or which supplements you take. It's also about how you feel when you wake up. Whether you're surrounded by people who uplift you or deplete you. Whether your mind is filled with noise or space. Whether your body feels like a safe home — or a battlefield.

And ultimately, that's what energy protection is: creating an internal environment where your body, mind, and spirit are no longer under siege.

It's reclaiming your space. It's learning to trust what you feel. And it's building a life that honors your energy — not as an afterthought, but as the foundation of everything else.

The Future of Health Is You

Becoming the Authority of Your Body

There comes a moment on every healing journey when you realize the most important expert you'll ever consult isn't found in a white coat, a wellness book, or a trending podcast — it's the voice inside your own body. This is not about dismissing medical professionals or scientific research. It's about recognizing that *you* live in your body, 24 hours a day. You're the one who feels the subtle shifts, the quiet warnings, the tug in your gut that something isn't quite right — or maybe finally is.

Yet for most of us, that inner authority was trained out of us early. We were taught to ignore it, override it, suppress it. If you had a stomachache before school, it was brushed off as nerves. If you said you were tired, you were told to push through. If something felt off but the test came back "normal," you were told it was all in your head. Over time, we learned to distrust our bodies — and in doing so, we lost touch with our most reliable compass.

Reclaiming that inner authority doesn't happen overnight. It's a quiet rebellion — not loud, not flashy, but deeply powerful. It starts with small decisions. Choosing to rest when your body whispers before it has to scream. Saying no even when you can't justify it on paper but feel it in your chest. Questioning what you've been told is "normal" if it doesn't feel right for *you*.

This is where the real reset begins — not just in diet or detox protocols, but in relationship. Your relationship with yourself. With your symptoms. With the stories you've inherited about what your body should be, look like, or be capable of. Becoming the authority of your body means recognizing that symptoms are not betrayals — they're messages. They're your body's way of alerting you that something needs attention. They're not the enemy; they're the entry point.

And yet, even as you begin to listen, the noise of the outside world doesn't go away. Every day, you're met with conflicting advice, marketing that preys on your insecurities, and systems that profit from your disconnection. This is why reclaiming your authority must be intentional. Because the default path is disempowerment. The default path says, "Someone else knows better than you."

But here's the truth most systems won't say out loud: your body holds a level of intelligence that no lab can replicate. That intelligence isn't mystical — it's biological, physiological, emotional, and yes, intuitive. It's what allows you to detect danger before it arrives. It's why you get a sense of who to trust without needing a spreadsheet. It's how you know when something is aligned — even if you can't articulate why.

The problem is, we've been conditioned to second-guess that intelligence at every turn. If your body says you're not okay, but a professional says you are, who do you believe? If a product makes you feel worse, but the label says it's "clean" or "healthy," do you trust your reaction or the branding?

This internal tug-of-war leaves many of us feeling stuck, unsure, and silently ashamed that we can't seem to "get better" the way we're supposed to. But what if the real issue isn't your body — it's that you've been trained to hand over the wheel, even when your internal alarm is blaring?

Trust is not something that clicks into place the moment you decide it's time. It's rebuilt, moment by moment, like a muscle that's been long neglected. And like any muscle, it can feel weak at first — shaky, unsure. But the more you practice listening, honoring, and responding with integrity, the stronger that inner authority becomes. It starts to drown out the noise. You stop needing everyone's approval. You begin making decisions not from fear of getting it wrong, but from the deep sense that your body knows what it needs, even if it takes time to interpret the message. You might begin to notice subtle shifts: your energy responds more quickly to the foods you eat. You sense tension building before a migraine ever arrives. You walk away from environments or people that leave you feeling drained — not because a study told you to, but because your body clearly said *no more*. This is self-leadership in its most grounded form. Not about control or perfection, but about partnership. You and your body on the same team, again.

Reclaiming this role as the authority doesn't mean you'll never need guidance or input from others. Quite the opposite. It means you'll know how to discern whose guidance truly aligns with your body's truth. You'll stop blindly outsourcing decisions. You'll start asking better questions.

You'll filter information through your own felt sense rather than defaulting to someone else's framework.

This also means making peace with complexity. The body doesn't speak in black-and-white terms. Healing is not linear. Some days, progress looks like more energy and clarity. Other days, it looks like stillness, discomfort, or even backtracking. That doesn't mean you're broken. It means you're learning to attune, to respond, to shift in real-time rather than forcing your body into someone else's blueprint.

You'll likely hit resistance — internally and externally. Not everyone around you will understand or support your choice to take your health into your own hands. There may be pushback, even ridicule. And there may be moments when old habits of self-doubt creep back in, whispering, *Who do you think you are to trust yourself this much?* That voice is not your truth. It's the echo of a system that profits when you stay small, silent, and confused.

But you are not confused. Not anymore.

You may not have all the answers yet — and that's okay. But you are no longer pretending that someone else has access to your body's wisdom better than you do. You are no longer ignoring the messages because they're inconvenient or don't fit into a spreadsheet. You are no longer afraid to pause, to feel, to choose differently.

This is what authority looks like. It's not loud or showy. It's steady. Rooted. Alive.

It's the way you begin to say no to the things that drain you — even when they're "normal." It's the way you reach for nourishment because it feels like care, not punishment. It's the way you notice, without shame, when something feels off, and give yourself permission to explore that without rushing for a fix.

And perhaps most importantly, it's the way you begin to trust that healing doesn't require you to become someone else — it requires you to come home to yourself. You're not a project to be corrected. You're a person to be reclaimed.

As you move forward, everything we've explored in this book comes back to this truth: you are the one who gets to decide how you live, how you heal, and how you thrive. Protocols can guide you. Research can inform you. Experts can inspire you. But only you can embody the wisdom that's been waiting all along — in your fatigue, your cravings, your tension, your joy.

This is your body. This is your life. And now, this is your authority. You're ready.

Living as Your Own Health Advocate

For too long, many of us have been trained to be passive participants in our own health journey. We sit in waiting rooms, hoping for answers. We accept rushed appointments and vague diagnoses. We fill prescriptions without fully understanding what they do. Somewhere along the way, the message was made clear: *the expert knows best — you just follow orders.*

But real, lasting health doesn't happen when you hand over your power. It begins when you become an active, informed, and unwavering advocate for your body — not just when something goes wrong, but every single day. Living as your own health advocate doesn't mean rejecting doctors or dismissing science. It means stepping into the driver's seat, asking better questions, gathering the right information, and taking ownership of the choices that impact your well-being.

Being your own advocate starts with presence. You can't make aligned decisions if you're disconnected from your own experience. Start by paying close attention to how your body speaks to you — not just through pain or symptoms, but through energy, sleep, digestion, mood, and cravings. These are not random annoyances to ignore or suppress. They're communication. They're clues. And when you learn to listen deeply, they tell you everything you need to know.

This kind of advocacy also requires education — not necessarily in the academic sense, but in becoming literate in your own physiology. You don't need to know every biochemical process. But you do need to understand the basics of how your body functions, what it needs to thrive, and how different systems — digestion, hormones, nervous system, detoxification — are interconnected. This knowledge creates confidence. It allows you to walk into appointments, conversations, or even health food stores with clarity, not confusion.

And with clarity comes discernment. You're no longer swayed by every new trend, influencer, or headline. You don't rush to try the latest supplement just because it's popular. Instead, you ask: *Does this make sense for me? How does this fit with what I know about my body, my history, and my needs right now?* This shift — from compliance to conscious decision-making — is a radical act of self-respect.

Of course, living as your own health advocate also means being willing to push back when something doesn't feel right. That could mean asking for a second opinion. It might look like requesting lab tests your provider initially dismissed. It could mean declining a medication, not out of fear, but because you're seeking a more root-cause approach. It might mean walking away from a practitioner who doesn't listen, believe, or support you.

These are not easy choices — especially if you've spent years internalizing the belief that speaking up is disrespectful, difficult, or dramatic. But advocacy isn't about confrontation. It's about alignment. When you know your body and you honor your intuition, you become much less willing to settle for answers that don't feel true or care that doesn't feel complete.

This doesn't mean going it alone. In fact, the best advocates know when and how to build a supportive team — professionals who welcome questions, who don't feel threatened by your curiosity, and who treat you as a partner in the process. These are the practitioners who respect your voice, your experience, and your right to choose. They exist — and your role as an advocate is to find them, not to shrink for the convenience of those who don't.

You'll also learn to advocate in the quieter moments — not just during appointments or emergencies, but in the grocery store, at the dinner table, in your own home. Every choice becomes an act of either depletion or nourishment. And when you're clear on what matters, even simple choices — what you eat, how you move, when you rest — become declarations of self-responsibility.

Over time, these small daily acts of alignment become the foundation for something deeper — a relationship with your body rooted in trust. This is not just about knowledge or strategy. It's about remembering that your body is not broken, not dumb, not defective. It's wise. It's responsive. And it wants to heal. When you start treating it like an ally instead of a liability, the entire way you move through life begins to shift.

You stop waiting to "get sick" before you act. You stop needing permission to rest, to nourish yourself, or to opt out of things that drain you. You become more attuned to your own boundaries — physical, emotional, and energetic. You stop outsourcing your well-being to external authorities who haven't walked in your skin, lived your stress, or felt your symptoms. And you start building the confidence to say, *I know something's off, and I'm not going to ignore it.*

That's not an easy stance to take in a world that's often quick to dismiss symptoms, minimize concerns, or funnel every issue into a one-size-fits-all protocol. It takes courage to believe in your experience, especially when it doesn't fit the textbook or when your labs are "normal" but you still feel far from well. Advocacy means holding space for the nuance — for what's not immediately obvious, but deeply real. It means giving your body a seat at the table.

Living this way also brings you face to face with your conditioning. So many of us were taught to be compliant, to be easy patients, to not question authority. We learned to suppress our discomfort, to be grateful for any care at all, even if it left us feeling unseen or unchanged. Undoing this programming takes time. You'll need to unlearn the reflex to apologize for asking questions. You'll need to practice trusting your gut, even when it contradicts what you've been told.

That trust grows the more you engage. Read. Research. Reflect. Don't just passively receive information — actively process it. Get curious. Compare sources. Ask practitioners why they're recommending what they are. Seek out others who've walked similar paths and can share what worked — and what didn't — for them. Build a personal framework that helps you make sense of what your body is experiencing. That framework is power.

And remember: advocating for your health doesn't mean obsessing over it. This is not about becoming hypervigilant or controlling. It's about awareness, not anxiety. It's about creating a baseline of support and clarity so that your energy can go toward living — not just managing symptoms or surviving. It's about choosing foods, routines, and environments that help you feel safe in your own skin, without perfectionism or fear.

Over time, you'll find that the voice that used to whisper *"something's off"* becomes louder, clearer, and more immediate. That's your inner advocate strengthening. You'll start making decisions not from desperation, but from grounded confidence. You'll ask better questions. You'll catch imbalances earlier. You'll respond rather than react. And when challenges do come — because life will still bring them — you'll navigate them with more agency and less fear.

Being your own health advocate is not a destination. It's a daily relationship with your body, your choices, and your sense of self-worth. It's an ongoing practice of self-leadership, especially in a world that often profits from your disempowerment. And it's one of the most radical, healing things you can do — not just for your physical health, but for your entire life.

You are not a passive observer of your own well-being. You are the primary steward. The more you listen, learn, question, and align, the more you begin to embody the truth that health isn't something you chase. It's something you create. And it begins with you.

Sustaining Your Reset for Life

You've done the deep work — peeled back the layers, rebalanced your gut, released toxins, rewired your habits, and stepped into a new level of awareness. But what now? The truth is, the reset isn't just something you complete and walk away from. It's not a cleanse, not a 30-day challenge, not a temporary fix. It's a recalibration of your relationship with your body and your life — one that only becomes more powerful the longer you stay in tune with it.

That's where sustainability comes in. Because healing isn't linear, and it certainly isn't static. You'll evolve. Your body's needs will shift with seasons, stressors, life stages, and even emotional breakthroughs. The goal now is not to stay rigid, but to stay present — to continue listening, adjusting, and honoring the intelligence of your body as it guides you forward.

Many people experience a kind of high after going through a reset. The clarity, the energy, the lightness — it feels like discovering yourself all over again. But over time, life will inevitably creep back in. Work deadlines. Family obligations. Late nights. Emotional stress. It's tempting to slowly revert to old patterns that once felt easier, more convenient, or more socially acceptable. And this is where so many people quietly lose their progress — not because they failed, but because they didn't have a framework for long-term integration.

To truly sustain your reset, you have to shift from motivation to embodiment. Motivation is a spark — it gets things moving. But embodiment is what carries you when the spark fades. It's what makes healthy living second nature instead of another item on a to-do list. It's when you no longer have to convince yourself to make aligned choices — you just do, because anything else starts to feel off.

That shift requires clarity about what truly supports you. By now, you've likely begun to recognize what drains you and what nourishes you — not in theory, but in your lived experience. Maybe certain foods fog your mind. Maybe late nights wreck your gut. Maybe certain environments or relationships make your chest tighten or your energy flatline. Honoring these observations isn't about restriction or paranoia. It's about alignment. When you choose what feels good because it *is* good — physiologically, emotionally, spiritually — you stop needing external rules to guide you.

But let's also be real: life is messy. You're not going to eat clean 100% of the time. You might skip your morning ritual. You might get overwhelmed and forget to breathe. That's not failure — that's being human. The key is not to spiral into shame or give up on yourself when that happens. The real work of sustainability lies in how quickly you *return*. How quickly you remember. How quickly you reconnect with the version of you who knows what you need and is willing to honor it.

The beautiful part is that every time you return, it gets easier. The reset becomes less of a conscious effort and more of a felt rhythm — your body starts craving what supports it. Your nervous system prefers peace over chaos. Your energy signals you when something is off. You become less tolerant of what once numbed you, less willing to override your intuition just to please others or keep up appearances.

So how do you create a life where your reset becomes your new baseline, not just a momentary upgrade?

It begins with building a flexible rhythm — not a rigid schedule, but a living framework that can bend and stretch without breaking. That means giving yourself room to adapt. Your daily rituals don't have to be identical every single day to be effective. Sometimes your morning walk might turn into a few minutes of deep breathing by the window. Sometimes your nourishing meal might come from a restaurant instead of your kitchen. What matters is that you're choosing with awareness, not falling into autopilot.

Awareness is the true foundation of sustainability. When you're aware, you're no longer making decisions from habit or pressure — you're making them from alignment. You know what makes you feel clear, grounded, and strong, and you know what pulls you off-center. That knowledge becomes a kind of internal compass you can rely on, even when life is busy, chaotic, or emotionally heavy.

And let's talk about consistency. There's a misconception that consistency means perfection — that unless you're doing everything right, every single day, you're failing. That belief is not only toxic, it's unsustainable. Real consistency is about coming back to yourself again and again. It's about staying in relationship with your health, even when you're tired or triggered or traveling. It's about making the next best choice, not the perfect one.

This mindset gives you room to be human. It lets you rest without guilt. It lets you eat the dessert without a side of shame. And most importantly, it lets you trust yourself. Because sustainability doesn't come from rules — it comes from trust. The more you trust your body to speak and yourself to listen, the more stable and lasting your reset becomes.

You can also create what I like to call anchor points — small, repeatable habits or rituals that help you reset throughout the day. These are less about performance and more about recalibration. A short grounding breath before meals. A check-in with your body before you open your laptop. A five-minute walk after lunch. These moments bring you back to your center, again and again, in a world that's constantly pulling you away from it.

Another important piece of long-term sustainability is community. Healing in isolation is possible, but it's harder — especially when the world around you reinforces disconnection, dysfunction, and distraction. Having even one person in your life who gets it — who values what you're building, who honors your boundaries, who speaks the same language of growth and integrity — can make all the difference. If you don't have that yet, seek it out. Whether it's a local wellness group, an online space, or simply someone you trust, connection is a nutrient too.

And finally, remember that the reset you've created is not about doing more. It's not about proving anything. It's about *being more* of who you already are. Health isn't something you chase — it's something you *return to*. Again and again, gently and honestly. You're not broken. You never were. You simply had to clear the noise, detox the confusion, and rebuild a relationship with yourself that's based on respect instead of neglect.

As you move forward, you may still stumble — and that's okay. Just don't stop listening. Don't stop choosing. Don't forget that you have already proven to yourself that healing is possible. Now your only job is to keep living like that's true — because it is. You've reset not just your body, but your identity. You're no longer someone hoping for health. You're someone living in it. And that changes everything.

www.ingramcontent.com/pod-product-compliance
Lightning Source LLC
Chambersburg PA
CBHW052210270326
41931CB00011B/2292